American Medical Association

Physicians dedicated to the health of America

Medical
Orthopedics

Conservative Management of
Musculoskeletal Impairments

D1004786

Rene Cailliet, MD

AMA Press

Vice President, Business Products: Anthony J. Frankos
Publisher: Michael Desposito
Director, Production and Manufacturing: Jean Roberts
Senior Acquisitions Editor: Barry Bowlus
Developmental Editor: Katharine Dvorak
Copy Editor: Kathleen Louden
Director, Marketing: J. D. Kinney
Marketing Manager: Reg Schmidt
Senior Production Coordinator: Rosalyn Carlton
Senior Print Coordinator: Ronnie Summers

Internet address: www.ama-assn.org

Additional copies of this book may be ordered by calling 800 621-8335. Mention product number OP857103.

ISBN 1-57947-409-8

Library of Congress Cataloging-in-Publication Data

Cailliet, Rene.
  Medical orthopedics : conservative management of musculoskeletal impairments /
  Rene Cailliet.
    p. ; cm.
  Includes bibliographical references and index.
  ISBN 1-57947-409-8
1. Orthopedics. 2. Musculoskeletal system—Diseases. I. Title.
  [DNLM: 1. Musculoskeletal Diseases—therapy. 2. Orthopedic Procedures—methods. WE 140 C1335m 2003]
RD731.C26 2003
616.7—dc21

2003000298

The authors, editors, and publisher of this work have checked with sources believed to be reliable in their efforts to confirm the accuracy and completeness of the information presented herein and that the information is in accordance with the standard practices accepted at the time of publication. However, neither the authors, editors, and publisher, nor any party involved in the creation and publication of this work warrant that the information is in every respect accurate and complete, and they are not responsible for any errors or omissions or for any consequences from application of the information in this book.

In light of ongoing research and changes in clinical experience and in governmental regulations, readers are encouraged to confirm the information contained herein with additional sources, in particular as it pertains to drug dosage and usage. Readers are urged to check the package insert for each drug they plan to administer for any change in indications and dosage and for additional warnings and precautions, especially for new or infrequently used drugs.

BQ76:03-P-077:07/03

Rene Cailliet, MD, is Professor Emeritus at the University of Southern California School of Medicine and a clinical professor at the department of Physical Medicine Rehabilitation at the UCLA School of Medicine. He has written eleven texts on musculoskeletal problems, which have been published in nine languages and sold more than 1.2 million copies.

CONTENTS

Medical orthopedics evolved from the premise that orthopedic problems are medical problems that respond to conservative nonsurgical interventions and should be addressed initially by the primary care physician. Most orthopedic problems conform to the following definition of *orthopedics:* "the branch of medical science that deals with prevention or correction of disorders involving locomotor structures of the body, especially the skeleton, joints, muscles, fascia, and other supporting structures such as ligaments and cartilage."[1] Orthopedics also is defined as "pertaining to or concerned with the treatment of disorders of the bones and joints, and the correction of deformities in general (orig. in children)."[2] Of these definitions, the former is more pertinent, as it deals with adults as well as children and deals with total "function" as well as "locomotion," which is defined as "the action or power, on the part of an organism or vehicle, of moving from place to place."[2]

Hence, I would formulate a newer definition of *medical orthopedics* as the science addressing "function" of the individual in the performance of activities of daily living that involve muscles, bones, joints, ligaments, and cartilage with minimal effort and absence of pain or discomfort. Intervention is not denied or demeaned, as it is important in correcting many deformities, but many impairments are correctable with conservative means pending their recognition. Normal function that is impaired, temporarily or permanently, must be addressed when recognized. This recognition is the intent of this text, as remedy is impossible without understanding normal function and why impaired function causes disability or the inability to function.

I have been a proponent of illustrating concepts of anatomical function in explaining the desired mechanical function, which is the basis of medical orthopedics—the restoration of normal functions by conservative medical means. Physical examination may need to be supplemented by radiologic diagnostic procedures, but a meaningful examination of appropriate history and visual-manual examination is usually adequate; hence I include illustrations to enhance the visual as well as manual examination outlined in this text.

Every musculoskeletal aspect of moving parts of the body must be addressed, as each plays a vital role in function. Treatment modalities must also be seen in this concept of restoring function. A large portion of this text (Chapters 10 and 11) also includes a discussion of pain and especially reflex sympathetic dystrophy, as both are too often neglected in the diagnosis and treatment of musculoskeletal impairments.

REFERENCES

1. Thomas CL, ed. *Taber's Cyclopedic Medical Dictionary.* 16th ed. Philadelphia, Pa: FA Davis Co; 1989.

2. Brown L. *The New Shorter Oxford English Dictionary on Historical Principles.* 4th ed. Oxford, England: Oxford University Press; 1993.

DISORDERS INDEX

Condition	ICD-9-CM 2003 Code	Page(s) in *Medical Orthopedics* Text
A		
Achilles bursitis or tendinitis	726.71	131–132, 133
Achilles tendon tear	845.09	132
Acute cerebrovascular disease (CVA)	436	170
Adhesive capsulitis of shoulder	726.0	82
Arachnoiditis	322.9	172
B		
Bone spur of heel	726.73	133–134
Brain infarct, unspecified	434.91	165
Brain infarct, embolic	434.11	165
Bucket tear of meniscus	836.0	145
Bunion	727.1	136–138
C		
Calcaneal bursitis, posterior	726.79	132–133
Calcaneal spur	726.73	133–134
Calcific tendinitis	726.11	77
Carpal tunnel syndrome	354.0	113–116
Causalgia	355.9	164, 166, 169, 178
Cerebrovascular accident (CVA)	436	170
Cervical lordosis	737.20	64
Cervical radiculopathy	729.2	170
Colles fracture, lower end, closed	813.41	112
Colles fracture, lower end, with open wound	813.51	112
Complex regional pain syndrome (CRPS)	337.20	94, 98–99, 163–192

Components of the Musculoskeletal System

In normal daily function, every component of the musculoskeletal system must be physiologically sound, as failure of any will impair total function. Thus, before the total structure and function of the musculoskeletal system can be evaluated, each of its components must be evaluated.

The musculoskeletal system is made up of ligaments, tendons, joint capsules, and muscles. The flexibility of each component will ensure the flexibility of the whole in the performance of the intended task. Limitation of one limits the range of the whole system and places unintended stress on the other tissues. In the evaluation of the impaired total function, the examiner must determine the normalcy of each tissue component. Most of these tissues play a passive role in the activity of the intended task.

Of the components of the musculoskeletal system, the muscles play an active role and must be judged by their strength, endurance, and length of contraction. All other related tissues influence these properties of the muscles and the role of these related tissues must be evaluated in any function. The nervous system has not been included as a component of the musculoskeletal system, as it will be discussed more fully in subsequent sections. With this total picture in mind, the various soft-tissue components will be discussed.

COLLAGEN

The collagen molecule is the basic structure that forms and supports all of the structures of the musculoskeletal system. Collagen fibers form the inner structure of dense connective tissue along with elastin and reticulum. The collagen fibers of connective tissues are involved in the epithelium, the nervous system tissues of the body, and the musculoskeletal system, all of which are the basis of medical orthopedics.

The term *connective tissue* is apt, as it implies a tissue that "connects" all tissues in a functional manner. In the 19th century, Virchow called collagen the "body excelsior" or "inert stuffing." Collagen fibers that form connective tissue are well structured for their purposes, which include:

- supporting specialized organs
- providing pathways for vascular tissues, nerves, and lymphatics
- permitting movement between adjacent tissues
- forming tendons and ligaments to facilitate and limit movement between contiguous structures
- attaching muscles to adjacent bones of an individual joint
- promoting circulation from arterioles, capillaries, veins, and lymphatics, thus assuring nutrition to these tissues.

Collagen fibers perform all of these functions by their architectural structure and their proportion to included elastin and reticular fibers. Their function is modified by the composition and hydration of the ground substance and the size and type of component collagen fibers.

The collagen fiber is a tropocollagen molecule arranged in a trihelical chain of amino polypeptides in which every third residue is the amino acid, glycine. These acids are chemically bound together with components of the matrix, which contains glycosaminoglycans, proteoglycans, and glycoproteins. There are currently many types of collagen—types I, II, III, IV, and IV—and each type contains subclasses. The type or types of collagen fiber are determined by the physical needs of the tissue in its function.

The component collagen fiber of connective tissue mechanically functions by its curled structure. In its passive phase it has a curvature that is equal to its function. Upon elongation, it uncurls and when the insertion upon adjacent bones shortens, the collagen fiber curls further.

Physiologic elongation (uncurling) from external stress on this viscoelastic tissue is called *creep*, which is defined as "a deformation that is gradual and under a constant load." It is termed *hysteresis* when the tissue loses energy from repeated loading and unloading. The term *anisotropy* implies strength and stiffness depending on the type, direction, and force of the elongation. Disruption of the amino acid chain occurs when the force exceeds physiological limits and neither recovery nor normal function is possible (Figure 1.1).

Collagen Fiber Normal trihelical amino acid chain has coiled structure that becomes uncoiled when passively elongated and more coiled when under no tension. Chains are connected by a bond at each intersection of the coils.

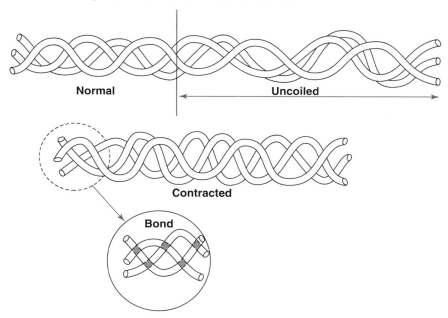

Temperature influences the viscoelastic properties of collagen, which, when added to the equation of force and speed of stress, may cause irrecoverable damage.[1]

Prolonged immobilization causes collagen fibers to fail to physiologically elongate and, within 4 weeks, decreases its physiological strength.[2] Severance of amino acid bonds is repaired by an invasion of fibroblasts that synthesize collagen but usually do so with fibrous tissue that forms an inflexible scar.

LIGAMENTS

Ligaments are uniaxial and able to resist loads in only one direction. The alignment of the component collagen fibers is parallel. With physiological loading, a ligament's strength increases, but excessive and rapid nonphysiological loading may cause failure. The characteristics of a ligament determine the type of injuries incurred, as shown in the following equation.

$$\text{Strain} = (\text{Increase in Length/Original Length}) \times 100$$

Normal loading (2% to 5%) of an isolated collagen fiber results in a deformation that returns to its resting length following release of the tension, whereas a strain of 7% to 8% causes a "plastic deformation," with failure to regain its normal resting length. Very-high-velocity stretching may overwhelm the ligament's viscoelastic properties and rupture the fiber bundles.[3,4]

Ligaments are passive structures that, along with the elasticity of the joint capsule, limit the degree of motion of joints. They function mechanically.

Proprioceptive nerves supplying joints, capsules, and the surrounding ligaments elicit impulses controlling the muscular reaction to prevent excessive motion of the joint (Figure 1.2). This reflex neurologic action becomes inoperative when the strain is rapid and unexpected. It has been shown that a ligament loaded to a sub-failure level and apparently grossly intact may become functionally deficient.[5]

Damaged ligaments heal by fibrous repair rather than by regeneration of damaged tissue. They heal in 3 phases:[3] (1) humeral response: coagulation, fibrinolysis, kinin, phagocytosis, mast cell degranulation, and prostaglandin release; (2) synthesis and deposition of collagen, which will contract in 3 to 14 days and continue for 6 months; and (3) remodeling, during which the collagen remodels to increase its functional capacity. This last phase may occur in 3 weeks and continue for up to 1 year.

TENDONS

Tendons are fibrous tissues that connect muscles to bones. Their inner structure comprises collagen fibers arranged in parallel, which gives them strength but little extensibility. They are plaited, in that they twine upon each other.[6]

Tendons are essentially avascular tissues that receive their blood supply from paratenon, a thin sheath that contains small blood vessels. Tendons vary in length and width depending on the muscle they serve and their desired function.

The cross section of the tendon is much less than the cross section of its muscle, hence the muscle fibers become concentrated at their site of insertion. Tendons are immensely strong. It has been estimated that a tendon with a cross section of 1 sq in is capable of supporting a weight of from 9700 to 18,000 lb.[7]

FIGURE 1.2

Neuromuscular Reaction to Joint Movement Proprioceptive impulses originating from joint structure activate neurons in dorsal horn of spinal cord, causing a reflex action on anterior horn cells (AHC), which moderate intrafusal and extrafusal fibers of muscles of that joint. Specific nerves serving this function are indicated. WDR indicates wide dynamic-range neurons.

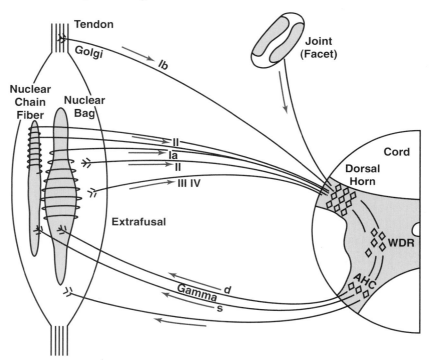

JOINTS

All joints move in a specific direction and require lubrication. A synovial joint is the space between 2 contiguous bones where each is lined with cartilage (Figure 1.3).

Joints are classified as congruous or incongruous dependent on the curvature of adjacent surfaces (Figure 1.4). This classification is important in the lubrication of the joint. A truly congruous joint cannot be lubricated, as any force on the joint compresses every aspect equally and thus lubricating fluid cannot flow. Self-lubrication depends on a wedge-shaped space where pressure at the apex forces fluid to the wider space.

FIGURE **1.3**

Typical Synovial Joint A synovial joint is the space between 2 contiguous bones where each is lined with cartilage. Capsule contains lubricant fluid created by unicellular synovial capsule and has an outer layer, or fibrous capsule, which limits degree of motion of that joint.

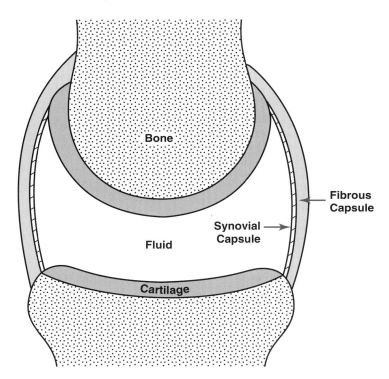

Joints begin to differentiate from primary mesenchyme in the human embryonic limb bud at 6 weeks and become defined as an articular structure coated with cartilage and with a capsule by 10 to 11 weeks. The nutritional pathways to adult cartilage change at maturity with closure of the epiphyseal growth plate and calcification.

JOINT CAPSULES

An articular capsule consists of a short sleeve of fibrous tissue called the *fibrous capsule*, which is lined with an inner synovial membrane called the *synovial capsule*. The synovial membrane folds over and approaches the articular cartilage. The synovial membrane is a thin

FIGURE 1.4

Congruity of Joint A, Congruous joint, where male portion rotates about axis (A) while the female portion (dotted shading) has equal spaces of joint a, b, c, and d. C indicates capsule; M, muscle actions on joint. B, Incongruous joint, where female and male surfaces are not symmetrical and male portion glides from (A) to (A) rather than rotates. C_1 indicates capsule.

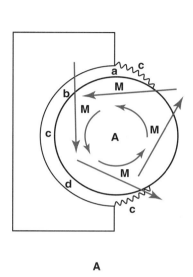

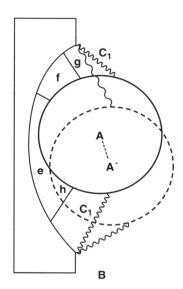

A   B

sheet of areolar tissue, which has a richness of blood vessels and lymphatic vessels.

The synovial membrane secretes synovial fluid, which lubricates the joint. This fluid is a dialysate of blood plasma plus a mucin of hyaluronic acid. This latter mucin adds viscosity to the synovial fluid and enhances its lubricant quality.

The folds of the synovial membrane contain fat at their attached borders and accommodate the changing size of the joint. The articular components of a synovial joint are incongruous, in that they do not fit each other reciprocally and are thus self-lubricating.[8]

CARTILAGE

Cartilage is a connective tissue that lines the ends of bones at each articulation. It does not have a blood supply, lymph vessels, or nerve endings.

Chondrocytes that form cartilage are considered to gradually decrease and to be totally terminated by the adult stage. More recent studies indicate that chondrocytes persist and continue to manufacture cartilage. Although there is no cell replication, chondrocytes remain metabolically active during the replacement of matrix. The thickness of cartilage gradually decreases with aging up to maturity, when it remains stable throughout remaining life.[9-12]

Water content is between 65% and 75% in normal cartilage matrix. The dry weight of cartilage is 50% collagen and proteoglycans. Cartilage collagen is type II, and the proteoglycans include glycosaminoglycans, chondroitin sulfate 5 and 6, and keratin sulfate that aggregate on hyaluronic acid. These form a proteoglycan molecule that is capable of binding large quantities of water.

There are 3 main types of cartilage: hyaline, fibrocartilage, and elastic. Cartilage lines the ends of bones in a joint, and its function is to repel or minimize compression, enhance freedom of movement with diminished friction, and furnish lubrication to that joint.

Hyaline Cartilage

Hyaline cartilage is clear, white, and translucent, and contains water. It contains collagen fibers so structured that they form coils similar to the springs of a mattress (Figure 1.5).

Nutrition of the cartilage is from the end blood vessels of the subchondral bones. The vessels do not enter the cartilage but release the nutritive fluid that is "imbibed" by the relaxing cartilage during its relaxed phase after compression (Figure 1.6).

Fibrocartilage

Fibrocartilage, in contrast, has the same structure, but the ground substance is less fluid and the collagen fibers are largely replaced by fibrous fibers. It is less compressible. Fibrocartilage replaces normal cartilage that has been damaged, as chondrocytes do not replace normal cartilage. Joints that are normally fibrocartilaginous have a more limited motion but are more stable.

Elastic Cartilage

Elastic cartilage contains a liquid matrix, and the enclosed fibers are elastic rather than collagen. Joints that contain elastic cartilage are joints needing greater flexibility and less stability.

FIGURE 1.5

Cartilage A, Cartilage contains a series of coiled collagen fibers forming "springs" within a matrix. Nutrition of matrix is diffusion from end blood vessels that terminate in subchondral bone. B, Any compression causes hyaluronic acid to be expressed from matrix-forming joint lubricant. Release of this pressure allows cartilage to expand and "imbibe" lubricating fluid, which becomes its nutrient. C, Gliding of adjacent cartilages is permitted by lateral angulation of coils and from lubricant.

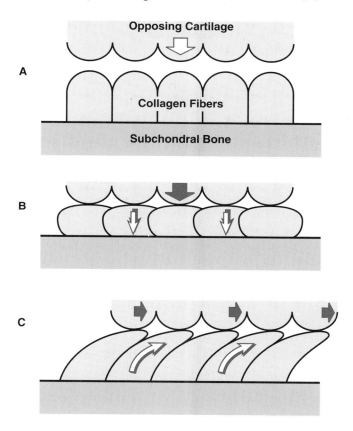

Any damage to cartilage causing ultimate degenerative joint disease occurs when the outer layers of the coiled collagen "springs" are damaged by shear forces (Figure 1.7).

Nutrition of Cartilage A, Osmotic pressure (OP). Cartilage covering subchondral bone in which terminal blood vessels that secrete nutritive fluid are located. B, External pressure (EP). Blood vessels (BV) within cortex of bone are end-organs whose fluid penetrates through subchondral bone (dark layer) into cartilage.

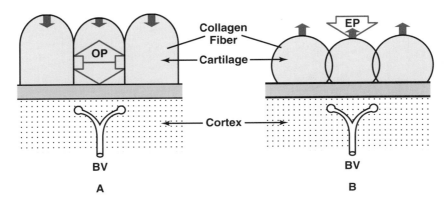

Shear-Force Damage to Cartilage A, Normal cartilage. B, Ends of "spring"-coiled fibers being damaged, with failure of coils.

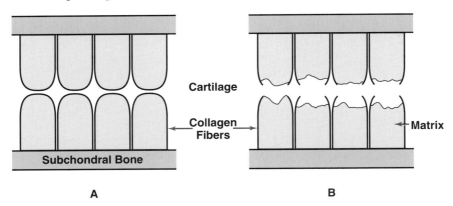

CONTROL OF NORMAL MUSCULOSKELETAL SYSTEM

Normal action of the musculoskeletal system is neurologically controlled. Action is initiated in cerebral cortex, where patterns are initiated and coordinated in brain stem, basal ganglia, and cerebellum and transmitted to spinal cord (Figure 1.8).

FIGURE 1.8

Neuromuscular System

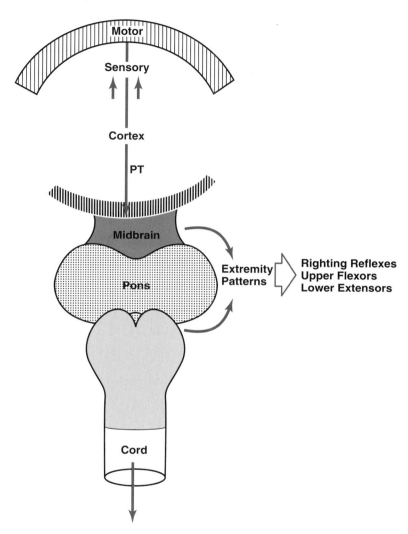

Motor fibers go to muscles for needed action. Muscles are moderated as to force and speed by spindle and Golgi systems. The central nervous system initiates the neuromuscular system function (the task), but the strength of the muscular contraction, its duration, and its length are determined by the intrafusal fibers (spindle and Golgi systems) (Figure 1.9).

FIGURE 1.9

Spindle and Golgi Systems

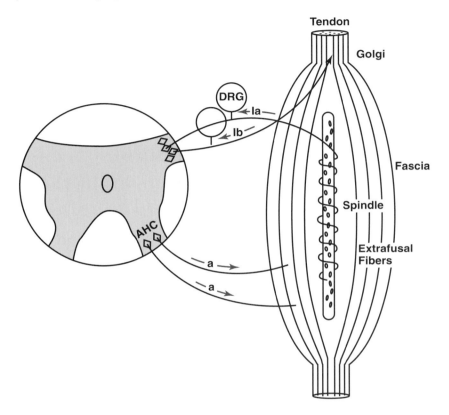

The spindle system consists of nuclear bag and nuclear chain fiber. Their sensory fibers II and Ia return to spinal cord, and their motor control is via gamma d and s fibers (Figure 1.10).

These symptoms are moderated by sensory proprioceptive impulses via Ib and Ia fibers that return to the spinal cord via the dorsal root ganglion. (Refer to Figure 1.9.) This reflex action is automatic and not totally under voluntary control.

Without muscles we cannot move or perform the activities of daily living, and without muscles the joints of the body cannot move. Voluntary skeletal muscles form 43% of the total body weight, and they connect with 2 bony points acting on joints. Muscle fibers are elongated cells of protoplasm containing several nuclei and a

FIGURE 1.10

Nerve Supply of Spindle System and Golgi Apparatus

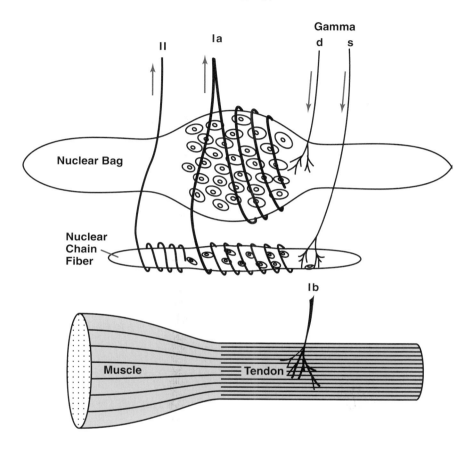

membrane. Each fiber ranges from 1 mm to 41 mm in length and is surrounded by loose areolar tissue, which permits the fibers to swell and assists in their gliding with minimal friction (Figures 1.11, 1.12).

The muscle fibers and their aponeuroses end into tendons. Muscles are contractile and vascular, whereas tendons are avascular and inelastic. A muscle contracts when the motor neuron impulse, originating in the anterior horn cell of the gray matter of the spinal cord, reaches the motor end plate of the muscle (Figure 1.13).

The mechanism by which a muscle contracts remains unclear, but there are numerous concepts proposed (Figure 1.14).

FIGURE 1.11

Organization of Skeletal Muscle Within a muscle fascicle are parallel fibers, each containing numerous fibrils. Fibrils are parallel strands of myosin and actin, which glide on each other during contraction.

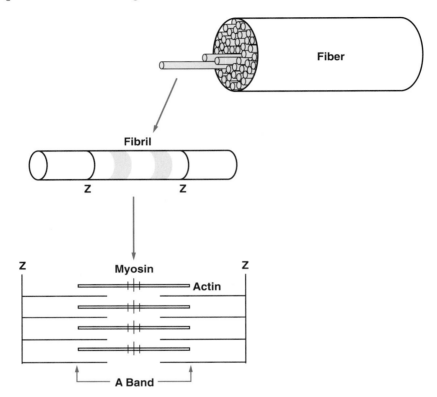

FIGURE   1.12

Contraction of Skeletal Muscle A, Relaxed muscle in which calcium (Ca) is retained in sarcoplasmic reticulum (Sarcoplasmic Ret). B, Thick lines are myosin, and thin parallel lines are actin, which glide on each other during contraction; this brings Z lines closer to each other. C, As muscle relaxes, calcium is pumped into sacroplasmic reticulum (downward arrows).

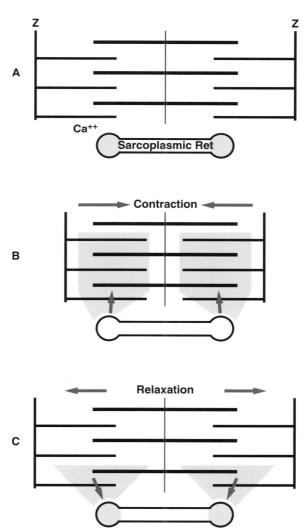

FIGURE 1.13

Motor End Plate Terminal motor nerve branches on a synaptic gutter, which resides under sarcoplasm (Sarc), where it deposits acetylcholine (Ach), which activates muscle contraction. This is subneural apparatus, which has small hair-like protrusions. MN indicate mitochondria; MY, myelin sheath of axon (AX); AX DIL, axoplasm dilatation.

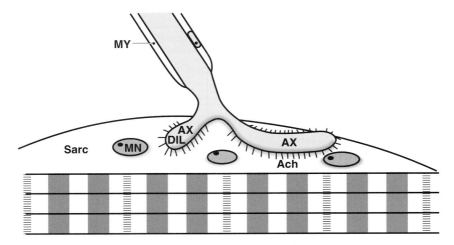

FIGURE 1.14

Mechanism of Muscle Contraction Once action potential of motor nerve reaches muscle, actin and myosin fibrils glide on each other, causing muscle to contract. A, Myosin molecule is a helix (2 protein chains) with a tail that ends in a "head." B, Myosin filament, made up of approximately 200 molecules, in a bundle alternating with parallel actin filaments that glide on each other. Actin is 2-strand helix, with one containing tropomyosin (darker strand). Troponin molecules attach to fibril. Actin filament and its troponin-tropomyosin complex are neutralized, and contraction begins. Contraction is assumed to occur as head of filament rotates about pivot site, causing "hinge" (tail-head filament of myosin molecule) to slide on actin filament. This is called *power stroke*.

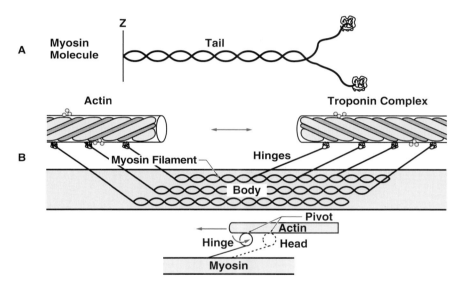

REFERENCES

1. Warren CG, Lehmann JF, Koblanski JN. Elongation of rat tail tendon: effect of load and temperature. *Arch Phys Med Rehabil.* 1971;52:465–474.

2. Noyes FR, Torvik PJ, Hyde WB, DeLucas JL. Biomechanics of ligament failure: II. An analysis of immobilization, exercise, and reconditioning effects in primates. *J Bone Joint Surg Am.* 1974;56:1406–1418.

3. Frank C, Woo SL, Amiel D, Harwood F, Gomez M, Akeson W. Medial collateral ligament healing: a multidisciplinary assessment in rabbits. *Am J Sports Med.* 1983;11:379–389.

4. Kellett J. Acute soft tissue injuries: a review of the literature. *Med Sci Sports Exerc.* 1986;18:489–500.

5. Youdas JW, Carey JR, Garrett TR. Reliability of measurements of cervical spine range of motion: comparison of three methods. *Phys Ther*. 1991; 71:98-104.

6. Basmajian JV. *Grant's Method of Anatomy*. 8th ed. Baltimore, Md: Williams & Wilkins; 1971.

7. Cronkite AE. The tensile strength of human tendons. *Anat Rec*. 1936; 64:173.

8. MacConaill MA. The movements of bones and joints: the synovial fluid and its assistants. *J Bone Joint Surg*. 1950;32:244.

9. Honner R, Thompson RC. The nutritional pathways of articular cartilage: an autoradiographic study in rabbits using 35S injected intravenously. *J Bone Joint Surg Am*. 1971;53:742-748.

10. Thompson RC, Robinson HJ. Articular cartilage matrix metabolism. *J Bone Joint Surg Am*. 1981;63:327-331.

11. Elliott RJ, Gardner DL. Changes with age in the glyosaminoglycans of human articular cartilage. *Ann Rheum Dis*. 1979;38:371-377.

12. Radin EL, Paul IL. A consolidated concept of joint lubrication. *J Bone Joint Surg Am*. 1972;54:607-613.

| 2

Vertebral Column

Of the many musculoskeletal conditions that cause severe economical distress as well as personal anguish, low back and cervical pain and impairment are predominant.

To fully understand pain and impairment from either the lumbar or cervical spine, the function of the spine must be understood and the functional impairment must be appreciated and addressed. The site of tissue damage causing nociception also must be ascertained.

The vertebral column, whether lumbosacral or cervical, is a mechanical structure composed of superincumbent functional units that consist of 2 adjacent vertebral bodies separated by an intervertebral disk and united by longitudinal ligaments, both anterior and posterior.

Posterior to the vertebral bodies are the lamina, pedicles, zygapophyseal joints (facet joints, or facets), transverse processes, and posterior superior spines. The bony structures of the lumbar and cervical functional units are similar in basic structure with only minor differences (Figures 2.1, 2.2, 2.3).

These superincumbent functional units are aligned in 3 physiological curves conforming to the center of gravity. These 3 curves form the cervical and lumbar lordosis and thoracic sacral kyphosis. The 3 curves are termed *posture*.

POSTURE

Roaf defined *posture* as "the position that the body assumes in preparation for the next movement," which involves balance, muscular co-ordination, and adaption.[1] Erect posture demands the minimum of muscular energy.

The "ligamentous spine" contains the structures that form the functional units. These include the intervertebral disks, which are

FIGURE **2.1**

Functional Unit: Side View "Functional unit" comprises 2 adjacent vertebrae separated by intervertebral disk. Pedicles (P) form margins of intervertebral foramen (F), through which passes the nerve root (NR) that immediately divides into anterior primary division (APD) and posterior primary division (PPD). Transverse processes (TP) and posterior superior spine (PSS) are sites of connection of ligaments and muscles.

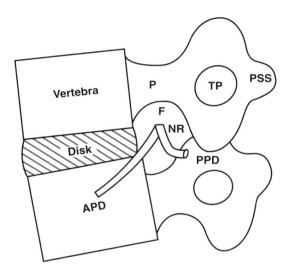

hydrodynamic structures that permit flexibility and withstand compression from gravity and especially from muscular contraction.

In the supine position the compressive load on the third lumbar disk has been considered to be 300 N. The load arises to 700 N in the erect position, and, in bending forward ahead of the center of gravity only 20 degrees, the load increases to 1200 N.[2]

Most studies of posture have been in the erect posture, both static and kinetic, with concentration on the lumbar lordosis and kyphosis.[3-6]

FIGURE 2.2
Functional Unit Seen From Above Vertebra forming a functional unit comprises disk with central nucleus (N) and surrounding annular fibers (AN), which are anterior in cervical unit. Posterior longitudinal ligaments (PLL) and anterior longitudinal ligaments (ALL) connect vertebrae. Posterior elements are pedicles (P), transverse processes (TP), and lamina (L) that connect, forming spinal canal (SC). Zygapophyseal joints (facets, F) are part of lamina. Erector spinal muscles (ESM) are shown, and dorsal root ganglia (DRG) of nerve root are within foramen.

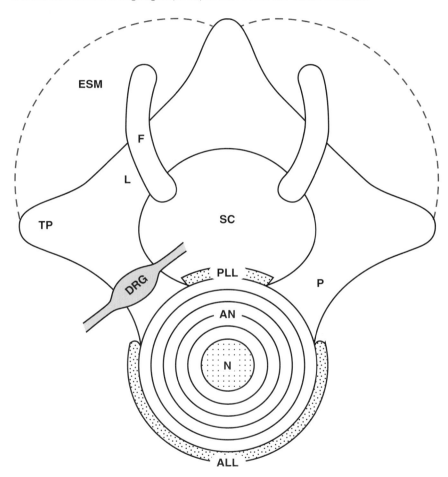

FIGURE 2.3
Cervical and Lumbar Functional Units A, Lumbar vertebra. Arrows show direction of herniation of nucleus (N) in injury. A indicates annulus; SC, spinal canal; LF, ligamentum flavum; PLL, posterior longitudinal ligament; and F, facets. B, Cervical vertebra with addition of uncovertebral joints (UVI), also called joints of Luschka. Arrows show direction of herniation of nucleus (N) in injury. F indicates facets.

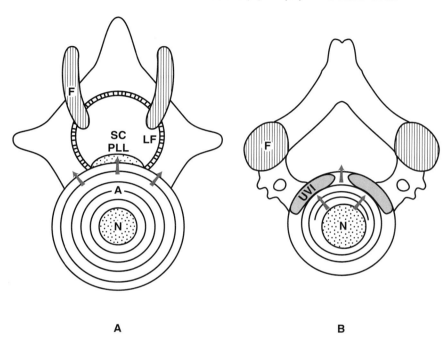

A   B

Seated Posture

Standing posture has been well documented in the literature over the centuries, but seated posture has not been that well documented, even though sitting posture has played an increasing degree of concern in therapists treating low back disorders.

The mechanical stresses upon the structures of the spine that relate to proper seating postures has had a long evolution, resulting in the current concepts of better seated postures. This aspect of ergonomics has not been adequately emphasized in the following definition of *ergonomics*: "the science concerned with how to fit a job to a man's anatomical, physiological, and psychological characteristics in a way that will enhance human efficiency and well being."[7]

Of the tissues that form the functional units of the lumbar spine that are stressed by postural seating, the following are most important in ensuring maximum comfort and minimal tissue damage:

■ Intervertebral disks,
■ Ligaments, and
■ Facets.

As seated posture is assumed to be static and not kinetic, the muscles of the trunk—the abdominal and the erector spinal muscles—are not directly involved, although they become secondarily involved.

Seated posture has been closely related to the structure and planes of the chair as well as the height of the seat from the floor and the functional purpose of the seated posture—professional or recreational. All of these factors play a role in seated posture.

Tissue Involvement of Seated Posture

With current concern about the role of the intervertebral disk in normal and pathological low back conditions, the effect of the seated posture on the disk is a major concern. This idea reached prominence by the studies of Nachemson[8] and Nachemson and Elfstrom[9] regarding intradiskal pressures and their dependence on changing postures, followed by similar studies by Sato et al.[10] These studies confirmed objectively that there were higher intradiskal pressures in the kyphotic posture than in the lordotic postures. However, the muscular effort in regaining lordosis neutralized that difference, indicating that seated posture in lordosis without any activity ensures the lowest intradiskal pressure in the seated position.[11-13]

In animal studies, a prolonged seated position with sustained kyphotic posture, ensuring sustained increased intradiskal pressure, showed increased degenerative changes in the disks.[8,9]

Increased intradiskal pressure also was noted in persons who leaned forward, forming a kyphotic posture with decrease in intradiskal pressure from assuming the lordotic curvature.

Reclining the backrest also reduced the intradiskal pressure, especially when lordosis was resumed.[12,13] More studies are needed to ascertain which postural lumbar curve is best and which chair inclination of the seat and backrest is more physiological. Currently the concept of maintaining lumbar lordosis during seated posture appears best suited for ergonomic reasons (Figures 2.4, 2.5).

FIGURE 2.4

Intradiskal Pressures in Kyphotic Posture Nucleus (N) migrates posteriorly during kyphosis, and posterior longitudinal ligament (PLL) undergoes strain. Besides increased intradiskal (D) pressure (vertical arrows), there is also shear stress (horizontal arrow). ALL indicates anterior ligament; V, vertebra.

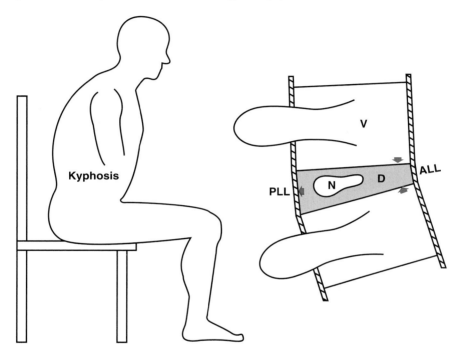

Effects of Posture on Facets

There also remains controversy regarding the pressure changes in the lordotic vs the kyphotic lumbar curves. Both impose pressure, as the role of the facets is to minimize shear stress and angulation occurs in both postures. Because both postures may injure the facets, the duration of the seated posture must be altered. Anterior disk narrowing causes greater impingement on the facets, so to minimize damage, frequent changes in seating posture must be assumed.

Posture has been discussed as possibly affecting the tissues within the functional unit—the disks, ligaments, and facets—so all must be evaluated.

FIGURE 2.5

FIGURE 2.5

Intradiskal Forces in Lordotic Posture In the lordotic posture the nucleus (N) migrates anteriorly away from the neural structures within the foramen but impinges upon the posterior annular tissues and the posterior longitudinal ligament (PLL), all of which contain nociceptive nerve endings.

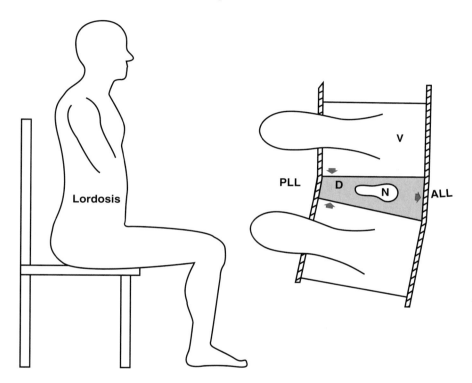

Management of Posture

Postural deficiencies may be due to a large number of causes including genetic factors, nervous system diseases, emotional status, disk diseases, and so on. Whatever the cause of postural deficiencies, which must be addressed, posture itself must also be addressed. Traditionally exercises, external supports, and even surgical intervention have been used and each plays a role in correcting the dysfunction.

Muscle Tone

The seeds of adult posture are sown in childhood, which is the time when posture must be addressed. This cannot be applied merely by prescribed exercises, which are not acceptable to most children for any period of time. Therefore, exercises, balance, and posture may be approached by athletic activities such as ballet and other organized sports activities such as rowing, basketball, and trampoline. Muscle tone, its control and integration, must thus be addressed and when a specific set of muscles are found to be defective they must be emphasized in the exercise program.

One exercise, in which the individual hangs by the arms applies traction to the trunk with elongation and also applies flexibility to the shoulder girdle. From this hanging position many trunk exercises can be implemented.

Splints or braces, which apply external force upon the trunk at appropriate levels, can correct the diagnosed abnormality, but this is a passive force that affects the spine during growth of the immature skeleton. But once the splint or brace is removed, the spine is allowed to resume its precast posture by the effects of gravity. Exercise must be instituted while in the support and especially after its removal.

Breathing and posture have not received appropriate attention. Holding a deep inspiration exercises the intercostal muscles as well as the abdominals and diaphragm. Balance, rhythm, and postural awareness must all be cultivated. Involvement of the arms is important in total postural treatment, as the arms exert external force upon the trunk. In the adult, Pilate's exercises emphasize this concept.

ANATOMICAL STRUCTURE OF THE VERTEBRAL COLUMN

There are 23 disks in the human spine, which account for 20% to 30% of its length. There are no intervertebral disks between the occiput, the atlas (C1), and the axis (C2). The sacral and coccyx vertebrae are fused.

The intervertebral disks are roughly cylindrical and of varying thickness. Each disk has a soft central nucleus surrounded by about 12 coaxial lamellae, each with a thickness of approximately 1 mm. The central nucleus is the element in the disk that distributes the compressive forces and separates the vertebral end plate.[14]

The fibers of the annulus surrounding the nucleus are collagen strands connected to adjacent vertebral end plates. In the nucleus, collagen fibers account for only 5% and are randomly dispersed compared with the outer annular fibers, which are well organized.[15,16]

FIGURE 2.6

Alignment of Annular Fibers of Typical Disk A, Alignments of sheets of collagen fibers. B, Effects of traction. C, Compression. D, Flexion. E, Shear. F, Normal alignment of individual annular sheets.

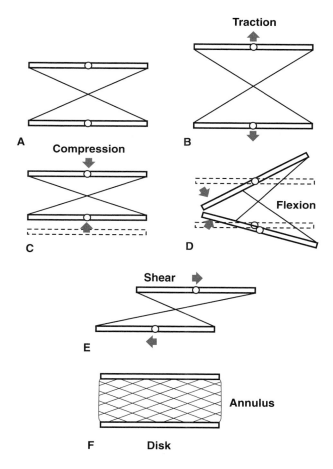

The annulus consists of sheets of collagen fibers that diagonally cross at approximately 30-degree angulation, and each sheet is aligned in opposite directions (Figures 2.6, 2.7).

The annular fibers are enmeshed within a matrix of proteoglycans containing approximately 88% water, hence its hydraulic properties.

As each collagen fiber unfolds, it has a limited extension, and when the tension is released, it recoils. Being of a viscoelastic material, these fibers have time-dependent mechanical properties.[16] The

FIGURE 2.7

Angular Variation of Annular Fibers A, Angulation of fibers in the outer sheets of the annulus (AN) (a-b). N indicates the nucleus of the disk; V, vertebra. B, Near the nucleus (N) the angulation of the fibers change (x-y). C, The change of angulation and length of the annular fibers during rotation. a-b > x-y indicates that the length a-b is longer than the length of fibers x-y, and c-d is greater than a-b during rotation.

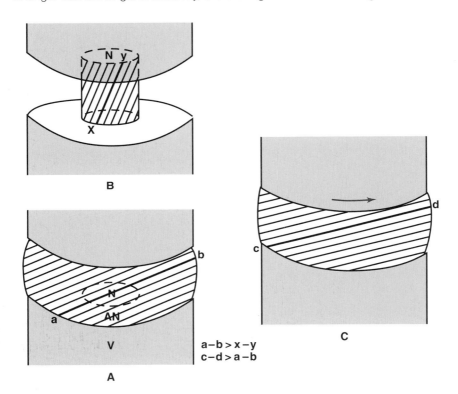

annular fibers of the disk are stretched when the functional unit of the disk is rotated, flexed, extended, and simultaneously compressed. The fibers of the annulus function to contain the nucleus as the unit deforms during motion. The outer annular lamellae provide strength during rotation and flexion or extension, whereas the inner lamellae suppress compression.

It is important to understand the normal structure and function of all of the components of the functional unit. When mechanical trauma exerts stress beyond the physiological limits of collagen fibers, the resultant elongation of these fibers results in their being torn or avulsed from their contact with the vertebral end plate.

FIGURE 2.8

Contents of Spinal Column Within spinal canal (SC) is the spinal cord (or *cauda equina*) with its dural sheath that contains spinal fluid (SF). Dura extends laterally into foramen, wherein is contained dorsal root ganglion (DRG), which is contained within nerve root (NR). Venous plexus (VP) drains epidural space. NR divides into posterior primary division (PPD) and anterior primary division (APD). PPD divides into muscular (Ms), joint (J), and skin (Sk) branches, and APD divides into motor (M) and sensory (S) branches. V indicates cervical vertebra.

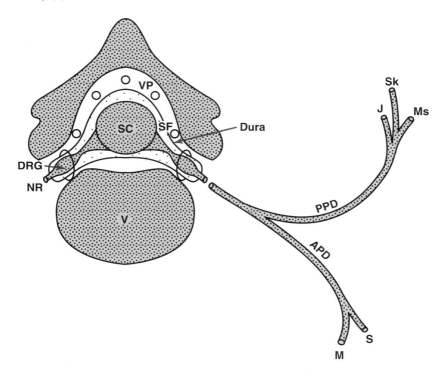

Disruption of the annular fibers results in the release of the nucleus from its central contained position enabling it to migrate outward through the tears. This condition is termed *internal* or *external herniation*, depending on the extent of the protrusion.

In addition to mechanical disruption of the fibers, allowing outward protrusion of the nucleus, chemical changes occur within the disk substances. This is a basis of nociception, which irritates nonmyelinated nerve endings in the nerve root dural sac, the posterior longitudinal ligament, and even the outer layers of the annulus.

Extrusion of disk material into the foramen or the spinal canal encroaches on adjacent tissues within the unit (Figure 2.8).

LUMBOSACRAL SPINE

The ligamentous spine is not considered as stable without the function of the erector spinal muscles and the abdominal muscles. Because these muscles are vital for the stability as well as for the specific motions of the spine and are incremental in malfunction and resultant pain, they should be thoroughly evaluated in both the lumbar and cervical spine.

Low back pain is so common a complaint that it has generated numerous medical articles as well as economic reports. At the 2000 International Forum for Primary Care Research on Low Back Pain in Israel, the comment was made that "researchers are on the verge of solving the back pain problem," but not all were in agreement.[17]

Gordon Waddell, a Scottish orthopedic surgeon, and his co-author[18] stated, "Don't turn a subjective health complaint into a medical condition." He implied that current medical thinking considers low back disability as a "disease," which is not in the accepted sense of the word.

Peter Croft from Britain noted about low back pain that "there is scant evidence that any form of medical treatment can alter the natural history of the prevalent condition over the long term."[19] In that same publication, Jeffrey Borkan, MD, the chairperson of the international forum, stated, "The traditional biomedical model of low back pain has generally proven to be a failure in primary care settings."[19] A biomedical model should be replaced by a model with impairment, not pain, being the primary goal of any intervention.

A "biopsychosocial" approach is gaining prevalence in the management of low back disorders. The psychosocial aspect of this approach gets precedence, and the "bio" aspect is neglected. Both are pertinent, however. The psychosocial aspect affects the "bio," but the "bio" aspect needs clarification. "Bio" must be understood to be the physical (mechanical) cause of dysfunction. Waddell and Burton[18] aptly state that low back problems "may not be gross anatomic disruptions but rather are a disruption of neuromuscular function and neurophysiology." How the psychosocial intervenes on the physiological remains unclear.

In an effort to internationally review all the related publications, the Cochrane Collaboration Back Review Group for Spinal Disorders was created in England in 1992. This group publishes its results to the following questions:[20]

- What works and what does not work in the treatment of back pain?
- What is the evidence and how strong is that evidence?
- How can a busy clinician distill this evidence and sort out the good?

Subgroups of the Cochrane Collaboration Group remain active in many countries periodically reviewing all pertinent literature.[1] All of these studies pertain to the modification of the incurred pain and its disability, but little attention is given toward understanding how the low back normally functions and how malfunction can be evaluated and altered.

The clinical biomechanics of the spine has been well documented, and research concludes that the impairment leading to the claimed disability is from impaired biomechanics. Of the tissues that are allegedly damaged and causing impairment, attention is directed to the intervertebral disk and its related tissues, but the specific relationship between the damage and the symptoms remains unclear.

The lumbosacral spine is a complex musculoskeletal structure that is made functional by an equally complex neurologic system. The neurologic sequence that activates the vertebral column, ensures its stability, and determines its precise movement originates in the cerebral cortex, where the intended task is determined at the precise moment by the person (Figure 2.9).

In early studies, Wilder Penfield postulated that all muscular actions were controlled by specific cells in the cerebral cortex when he stimulated individual neurons in the premotor cortex and elicited a specific muscular response.[21] Later studies have refuted individual muscle response and have postulated that all muscular movements occur in patterns.

Motor activity occurs in 2 stages: planning and execution. In either stage the activation phase of the action is planned in the upper neurologic system—the cortex, midbrain, basal ganglia, and cerebellum—but the details of torque and force are moderated in the muscular system by the spindle and Golgi systems. The question, "Does the brain represent movement?" has been raised by numerous neurophysiologists, but the question remains unanswered.

The ligamentous spine is known to be unstable at loads less than half the weight of the body; when those loads are augmented by weights in the hands, the spine deviates from the center of gravity.

FIGURE 2.9

Neurologic Sequence of Spinal Activity All intended movements to perform a desired task originate in cerebral cortex (?). All resultant neuromusculoskeletal motions occur as patterns, which are engrained in cortex, midbrain, basal ganglion (BSL GGL), and cerebellum (Cereb). From there, impulses are transmitted through spinal cord to extrafusal muscle fibers. Muscle contractions are moderated by spindle system (SPL) and Golgi apparatus (GLG) in determining strength, tension, and rapidity of action. Muscles move joints of the spine: disks and facets.

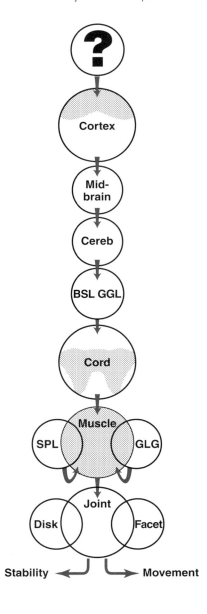

FIGURE 2.10

Ligamentous Spine Lumbosacral spine supports 2 inflexible systems: thoracic spine, which is made inflexible by ribs; and pelvis, which articulates between the 2 femoral heads. Figure at right shows instability of the 2 segments balanced by a flexible rod: lumbar spine. CG indicates the center of gravity.

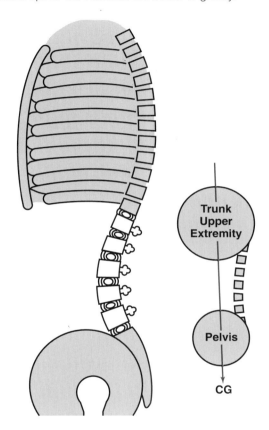

The mechanical support of the ligamentous spine is considered the "passive subsystem," which buckles when the superimposed load, termed the *critical load of the spine*, is exceeded (Figure 2.10).

The muscular system is considered mandatory to sustain the erect spine. The extrafusal muscle fibers with their fascia and tendons are a vital portion of the stable spine. There is a feedback system in which the proprioceptive impulses from the disk, facets, ligaments, and tendons activate and modify the muscular reaction that is moderated by the intrafusal system: the spindle and Golgi systems (Figure 2.11).

FIGURE 2.11

Intrafusal Control of Neuromusculoskeletal System Proprioceptive impulses from joints activate spindle and Golgi systems controlling muscular system.

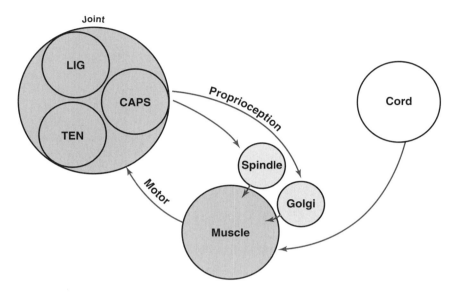

The muscular system presents a formidable aspect of low back disorders, in that its malfunction results in impaired flexibility, loss of range of motion, painful tension, and nodularity within the muscle tissue, as well as impairing all of the other ligamentous aspects of the spine: the disk, facets, and ligaments. None of these muscular conditions has been fully explained until the proposed concept of C. Chan Gunn.

Gunn postulates that most painful and impairing conditions of the vertebral column are the sequel of "spondylosis," which may be dormant and asymptomatic until a force impairs the stability when a "radiculopathy" results.[22] This *radiculopathy*, termed by Gunn, is a motor mononeuropathy in which the motor fibers are irritated at the foramen from a spondylosis resulting from disk degeneration.[23] The spondylosis mentioned by Gunn is a slow, gradual disk degeneration. It remains silent and asymptomatic but mechanically and gradually narrows the foramen, allowing little room for migration of the emerging nerve root (Figure 2.12).

The narrow foramen, which contains a nerve that has been irritated from minor traumas, now becomes compressed, which causes

FIGURE 2.12

Spondylosis Radiculopathy of Gunn As disk space narrows, vertebrae (V) approach (open arrows), narrowing foramen (solid arrows) through which nerve, motor, and sensory roots emerge. Compression on larger myelinated motor nerve root causes muscle to contract and remain contracted until released by intramuscular stimulation.

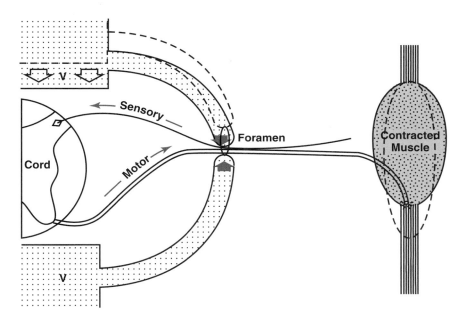

discharge of the irritated but previously normally functioning nerve. Cannon and Rosenblueth proposed a law (called Cannon's law) that postulates: "When in a series of efferent neurons a unit is destroyed, an increased irritability to chemical agent develops in the isolated structure or structures, the effects being maximal in the part directly denervated."[24] This showed that muscles, both striated and smooth, develop sensitivity. The muscle area enlarges and is very sensitive to acetylcholine.

This change (hypersensitivity) is noted within a matter of hours after administration of acetylcholine and reaches its maximum within a week. It is important to understand that actual physical interruption is not necessary for "denervation hypersensitivity" to develop. Minor degrees of damage can destroy the microtubules within the nerve axons, leaving the nerve still able to conduct nerve impulses.[8,9]

The resulting segmental contraction of the muscle from the supersensitive mononeuron of the specific nerve root now causes restriction of motion, localized pain, and tenderness of the muscular nodule, which remains until the cycle is interrupted. Palpation of that specific muscle segment early in the radicular history becomes a confirming diagnostic sign, and elimination of this nodule by dry needling becomes therapeutic.[10] Much of this law may be considered as speculative at this stage, but there is increasing evidence of its validity and further study will clarify its significance.

Static Spine

Clinically the erect static spine usually poses no great concern other that in people who spend much of their day in the erect posture. The medical history makes it clear, and the results of the examination confirm the basis of the impairment. An excessive lordotic posture is usually the culprit in static low back discomfort, which can be reproduced clinically by passively and actively creating an excessive lordosis. Radiologic studies may confirm excessive angulation of the lower spinal segments with facet narrowing and even reveal a degree of spondylolisthesis.

Kinetic Spine

Most patients with low back disorders allegedly sustained their "injury" from the performance of an activity that they recall and report. When such a history is carefully reviewed, most cases of low back pain can be considered as having resulted from a deviation from normal kinetic function. ("Kinetic" comes from the Greek word *kinesis*, which is defined as "consisting of motion.") In the performance of a physical task, there is deviation of the body from the center of gravity, with the body having assumed a position ahead of the center.

All of the tissues of the back that maintained the erect static posture are now altered in their function. The muscles that were contracting isometrically now become isokinetic. The abdominal muscles that were functioning to maintain stability now become flexors and rotators. The extensor muscles that were stabilizers now become decelerators that elongate with appropriate speed and force to accomplish the intended task.

The disks, the facet joints, and their capsules of the ligamentous spine now deform within their physiological limits. As the spine

FIGURE 2.13

Kinetic Functional Unit Functional unit is shown from the side. Intervertebral disk (IVD) is located anteriorly. In flexion (F), interspinal ligament (ISL) and superior spinous ligament (SSL) elongate. Superior vertebra shears forward (S to SH).

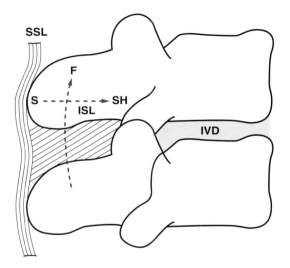

flexes, the vertebra of each functional unit of the spine flexes, gliding slightly forward within the limitations of the annular fibers, the long ligaments and the capsules of the facets (Figure 2.13).

Any kinetic action of the spine demands a complex neuromusculoskeletal kinetic action. The components of the ligamentous unit are moved appropriately and anatomically within normal limits. If any of these motion components are violated or performed in an abnormal manner, dysfunction results, with injury to one or more of the components of the functional unit. Low back disorder results, with impaired function and pain.

The medical history depicts the action that precipitated the disorder, and the examination attempts to confirm the specific tissue of the functional unit that has caused the impairment. The offending action identified from the history is often a repetitive motion that causes fatigue, distraction, and/or boredom, with inattention resulting in inappropriate movement. This inattention from fatigue or boredom also may cause a misinterpretation of the weight of the task or the distance to be moved. The subsequent action on the functional unit results in mechanical damage to one of the tissues of the unit.

FIGURE 2.14

Tissue Sites of Nociception Accepted sites of nociception within a function unit. 1 indicates dorsal root ganglion of nerve root; 2, facets (F); 3, outer annular fibers of intervertebral disk (D); 4, posterior longitudinal ligament; 5,vertebral artery and its sympathetic nerve supply in cervical spine; 6, erector spinal muscles (ESM); 7, posterior spinous ligaments; V, vertebra; L, lamina; P, pedicle and SC, spinal cord.

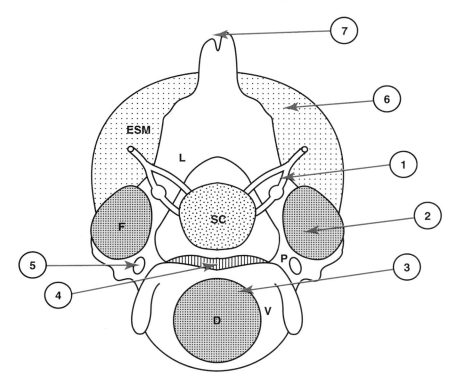

Tissue Sites of Nociception

The injured tissue releases nociceptive chemical elements that result in pain, which further alters the needed normal neuromuscular kinetic function. The sites of nociception from the injured tissue of the functional unit are shown in Figure 2.14.

Injury to any of these nociceptive sites causes "protective muscular reaction" termed *spasm*. Clinically, spasm is present and causes impairment as the muscle shortens and prevents elongation, inhibiting any movement of the ligamentous spine. When prolonged, spasm causes muscle ischemia, which becomes a nociceptor.

In the neuromuscular concept of spasm, impulses from an inflamed joint are transmitted to the dorsal horn neurons of the spinal cord, which are then transmitted to the wide dynamic-range neurons (WDR) and then to the anterior horn cells that motor the extrafusal muscle fibers. Impulses also are transmitted via gamma fibers to the intrafusal fibers, which causes failure to adequately monitor muscle contraction. Persistent contraction of the extrafusal fibers causes ischemia and excessive lactic acid. These nociceptive elements are transmitted back to the spinal cord via II, III, and IV sensory fibers, causing a vicious cycle with persistent muscular contraction referred to as spasm. Those concepts do not refute the concept of Gunn, as all of the efferent and afferent fibers shown are present in the nerve root that emerges via the foramen.

Ischemia as a nociceptor has been discussed in the literature.[25] The normal biological substances that act on vessels and nervous structures are known as *vasoneuroactive substances* (VNS); they cause only local or general damage when they increase in concentration. Among the VNS are catecholamines, serotonin, histamine, kinins, and prostaglandins. Ischemia provokes a local activation of kinin and serotonin. Ischemia from prolonged intense muscular contraction releases 5-hydroxytryptamine and bradykinin from platelet and plasma kininogen, which stimulate the pain receptors.

It is also of interest and significance that supersensitivity (Gunn's concept of "prespondylosis") from denervation reduces the total collagen in skeletal tissues. The replacement of collagen is with collagen of fewer cross-links, which makes it weaker than normal collagen tissue. This weakened collagen is a substance of the disk annular fibers, tendons, and ligaments, which is ominous in low back disorders.[26]

Spinal Stability

Spinal stability, which is not present in the ligamentous spine, has been well established as requiring appropriate muscular strength and endurance. The muscles of the trunk affording this stability are the transversus abdominis and the erector spinae multifidus.

Prolonged posture and repetitive flexed positions elicit reflexive contraction of the multifidus muscles. This contraction "desensitizes" the mechanoreceptors of the facets, ligaments, and disk annulus within a 3-minute period, causing a loss of muscle contraction and thus a loss of stability. This adds a temporal factor in ergonomics so that fatigue must be avoided in daily tasks by requiring periodic breaks.

Before any attempted activity, the static spine, which is made stable by its viscoelastic support and its isometric muscular component, must augment this static support in preparation of the contemplated kinetic action. The mechanoreceptors of the spine signal the musculature of the precise muscular contraction needed for the intended task: the force, speed, and length of muscular contraction.

Any deviation from this complex motion, the proper precedent static posture with its isometric muscular contraction followed by the appropriate kinetic (neuromuscular) activity of the spine for the intended task, results in injury to the end-organs. The disks, the facets, their capsule, and/or the ligaments are the end-organs affected.

These end-organs must be structurally and functionally adequate to undergo the required physiological motion. The disks must compress, rotate, flex, and glide to the appropriate degree of motion to accomplish the task intended. As all functional units of the lumbosacral spine move in a concerted motion, each unit—the disks, the facets, their ligaments, and the paraspinous muscles—must perform its part of the motion.

Excessive or faulty motion of the functional unit causes damage to one or more of the involved tissues, with resultant nociception impairment and pain. In an inadvertent motion the annular fibers of the disk may be elongated beyond their physiological limits and either tear or avulse from the attachments to the vertebral margins.

Rotational forces rather than mere compressive forces have been noted to cause the most damage (tearing) to the annular fibers. Tearing of annular fibers permit herniation of the otherwise contained nucleus, allowing the nuclear matrix to bulge through the annular tear. Initially this constitutes an "internal" herniation, which may not be visible on magnetic resonance imaging (MRI) studies but causes several pathological aspects, resulting in pain and impairment. The tear causes chemical breakdown of the matrix, releasing nociceptive elements that may irritate the sensory nerve fiber endings. This chemical breakdown is essentially breakdown of the disk mucopolysaccharides, releasing kinins, nitric acid, prostaglandins, and other products.

Tearing of inner annular fibers results in the other outer annular fibers having to bear the brunt of restraining the nucleus. This causes some bulging of the outer annular sheaths against the longitudinal ligament and even the content of the foramen: the nerve roots and their dural sheaths. Either of these internal herniation sequelae can result in the clinical manifestation of internal disk herniation: pain, secondary spasm, and restricted spinal motion (Figure 2.15).

FIGURE 2.15

Internal Disk Herniation Tearing of disk annular fibers allows nucleus (N), which is under intrinsic pressure to herniate (arrow) into spinal canal (SC). Outer annular fibers bulge outward under this pressure against dorsal root ganglion (DRG) and/or posterior longitudinal ligament (PLL).

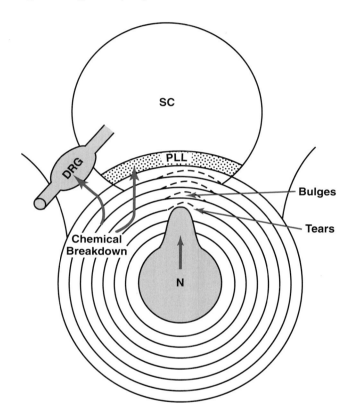

If the herniation is posterolateral against the dorsal root, ganglion pain and impairment occurs down the leg in the dermatomic region. If, however, the pressure is against the posterior longitudinal ligament, pain is noted in the midline of the low back and accentuated by trunk flexion, which causes stretching of that ligament.

Pressure alone against the dorsal root ganglion of the nerve root or the posterior longitudinal ligament without accompanying chemical irritation does not result in pain but merely paresthesia. Only the nerve tissues that are chemically inflamed respond to compression with pain.

As the disk sustains annular tears, there are simultaneous changes in the matrix, which impair its hydrodynamic function and diminishes its stability. With impairment of the hydrodynamics of the disk, the posteriorly placed facets, whose separation depends on the intactness of the disk, also lose their functional integrity. Their capsule and cartilage undergo damage.

The facets have large numbers of sensory nerve endings subserving proprioception and nociception, which become impaired when compressed. Facet inflammation causes pain on low back extension, especially when there is simultaneous lateral flexion to the side of the pain.

If an annular tear is posterolateral, it encroaches on the nerve root, causing radiating pain into a dermatomic area, and there will be limited ability to keep the leg straight while raising it. There will be radiating pain, impaired sensation into the dermatomic areas, and muscle weakness in the myotomic regions of the specific nerve or nerves involved. These are determined by a careful neurologic examination.

LOW BACK DISORDERS

History

The patient usually presents with the complaint of pain in the low back and not a loss of any specific function. The pain site usually is not specifically delineated as to the precise tissue site but rather merely to the low back area. The description of the pain also does not specify the neurologic basis of the tissue site, but muscular reaction is the basis of impairment.

The person initially may assume an antalgic posture created by the muscle spasm, which diminishes the spine flexibility and prevents motion in all directions, definitely in flexion and reextension. This "antalgic" characteristic of the spine shows the loss of the physiological lordosis, with the spine assuming a straight configuration.

Movement in any direction—flexion, extension, lateral flexion, and/or rotation—is limited. If there is unilateral spasm, a "functional" scoliosis occurs, causing the spine to be lateral to the center of gravity. Muscle tenderness, which may occur, is probably from the ischemia that results from the sustained muscle protective contraction (spasm). The ligamentous tissues of the spine, which are under the control of the muscular system, malfunction, causing the symptoms and impairment. These tissues now become the focus of the evaluation.

Biopsychosocial Aspects of Low Back Disorders

The psychological factors that influence the pathomechanism of low back pain need clarification as to whether they are contributory or merely responsive. "Contributing" to low back disorders implies that the normal biomechanical function is misdirected because of psychological factors. Some of these factors have been mentioned, such as anxiety, impatience, depression, and anger.

Fear

Fear is a major psychological factor. It is well accepted and documented that fear of recurrence greatly influences low back disorders (Figure 2.16). Such fears must be realized and addressed in any patient who is disabled due to a low back disorder, as fear can increase the degree of impairment as well as magnify the degree of pain.

Fatigue

Fatigue is also a prominent cause of low back disorder. This physiological aspect of neuromuscular skeletal function is revealed by obtaining a proper history:

- Was there preexisting fatigue from repetitive motion of flexion and/or lifting?
- Were there sufficient breaks in the daily activity to prevent fatigue and boredom?
- Were there extraneous factors, such as personal or job stresses, that could have impaired proper body mechanics?
- Was the person in reasonable physical fitness having good flexibility as well as good abdominal and extensor muscle strength of the low back?
- Were proper ergonomics practiced or even understood?
- Was there a previous painful episode? If yes, what was considered responsible, how long did the episode last, and how was it treated?
- What does the patient consider the cause, the basis of the current condition, and how important is the condition as to recovery and ability to resume normal functions?

There are numerous causes of low back pain and dysfunction, which include:

- Mechanical low back impairment,
- Herniated lumbar disk,
- Spinal stenosis,

FIGURE 2.16

Influence of Fear on Normal Neuromuscular Function Neurophysiological mechanism of function is influenced by fear as a concept of significance (at right) and from memory of other pain syndromes (at left). Arrows with Rx indicate sites on therapeutic intervention.

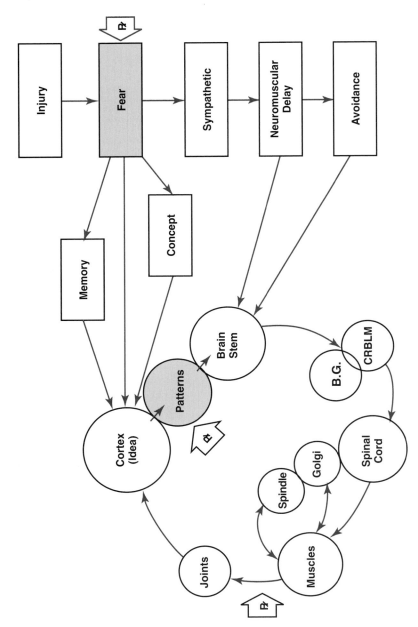

■ Spondyolisthesis, and

■ Musculoskeletal disease, which involves the low back among other sites.

Each condition presents specific facts of history as to the site of pain and mechanisms of aggravation and also present variations upon physical examination that denote the exact cause. Many rely upon radiological examinations for specification of the specific cause.

Physical Examination

The medical history has implied the action that precipitated the low back disorder as well as the patient's understanding of "what happened." The physical examination must evaluate the physical findings that objectify the subjective history. Which motions are denied the patient or elicit pain?

The following questions are answered after an appropriate examination:

■ Is there limited flexibility (and which direction)? Which motion is avoided or unable to be performed, and when it is performed, where is the pain located?

■ Is there local tenderness of the paraspinous muscles, and is the reaction of the patient appropriate or exaggerated?

■ Can the patient perform straight-leg raising on both sides, and is the motion reinforced with simultaneous neck flexion or ankle dorsiflexion?

■ What are the results of dermatomic testing with cotton, pinprick, and vibration tuning fork?

■ What are the results of muscle testing of each myotome?
   a. Ankle dorsiflexion, big toe flexion, and extension (S1 and L5)
   b. Musculus gastrocnemius: patient stands up on the toes of each foot repeatedly (S1)
   c. Reflexes: ankle jerk and knee jerk to reflex hammer

■ Are there tenderness and/or nodularity of the involved muscle or muscles considered restrictive and painful?

Specific Conditions

Mechanical low back pain and dysfunction merely impair low back function without radiculopathy. There is pain located in the low back and limited flexibility with any attempt at exceeding that limitation, causing pain and guarding. Radiological studies may not be diagnostic and the neurological examination is within normal limits.

If there is suspicion of a disk herniation, there is subjective radicular symptomatology—pain, numbness, and/or paraesthesia felt in the lower extremity in a dermatomal area. The radicular component of the syndrome is confirmed by the presence of pain aggravation upon straight leg raising (as compared to the opposite side) that is further aggravated by simultaneous nuchal flexion and/or simultaneous ankle dorsiflexion.

The neurological examination further confirms the presence of nerve root entrapment, as well as designates the spinal area. A disk herniation at the L5-S1 spinal level is noted to have a diminished and even absent ankle tendon reflex and weakness and/or fatigue of the gastrocemius muscle group. The specific muscles within the myotome may show weakness of the ankle evertors. There is impaired sensation to light touch and pinprick of the S1 dermatome. There is weakness and fatigue of the gluteus maximus hip extensor.

Herniation of the disk between the lumbar 4 and lumbar 5 vertebra implicates the L5 dermatome, causing weakness of the great toe extensor and flexor but sparing of the reflex change.

Herniation of the disk between the L3-L4 vertebra often does not produce a positive straight leg raising but does cause limited and painful femoral nerve stretch, which is done with the patient in the prone position and the leg hyperextended.

Radiologic Studies

Routine x-ray films are usually of no great diagnostic value after a trauma unless a fracture or dislocation is suspected. Computed tomography (CT) and MRI studies are indicated when there is need for anatomical confirmation of the condition that persists beyond an expected duration and after a reasonable period of therapeutic intervention when surgical intervention may be indicated.

Magnetic resonance imaging is currently used to diagnose the presence, level, and degree of disk herniation, but an abnormal finding that does not confirm an abnormal physical examination is not considered a valid reason to imply the diagnosis.

Treatment

Management of low back disorders can be divided into three phases: acute, recurrent, and chronic. All three have some similarities, but all have basic differences.

The first approach in management of low back disorders is to inform the patient of the mechanical aspect of the impairment and not imply that a "disease" is present. The mechanical cause of the patient's symptoms must be addressed in clear, understandable terms. Unfortunately, terms such as *degenerative, arthritis, disk ruptures*, and *sciatica*, are used by practitioners and may not be understood by the patient. The mechanical basis of the symptoms and impairment is lost to the patient and to the practitioner with the resultant concept of "disease" replacing the concept of transient physical impairment.

The psychological factors that have been known to aggravate the condition and make it intractable are put into place by this cavalier approach. With explanation and thus reassurance that the condition is mechanical and treatable allays the component of fear.

Whether acute, recurrent, or chronic, there are general factors that must be implemented in the treatment of low back disorders:

- Immediate reassurance of the patient as to the mechanical aspects of the condition and the avoidance of implementing this as a "disease."

- Furnishing a diagnosis based on explaining the mechanism of the impairment and the pain rather than using terms such as *disk disease, disk herniation, sciatica,* and so on (but if these are confirmed findings, their significance and meaning must be explained to the patient).

As pain is a major concern to the patient, its site of causation and its significance must be clarified. Relief of the symptoms of pain can be addressed by the use of oral analgesics such as nonsteroidal anti-inflammatory drugs (NSAIDs). Local ice application upon the low back area for 20 minutes for 48 hours then application of hot packs has value alone and in conjunction with other modalities. Their benefit as well as decreasing pain allow the implementation of activities such as exercises, which must be instituted early, as exercises have value in regaining flexibility and muscle tonus that is necessary for spinal stability. Exercise not only improves the mechanical stability of the low back but also permits resumption of normal activities of daily living.

An article in *Spine*[27] concluded that a wraparound heat pad to the entire low back for 3 to 4 days was more effective than oral anti-inflammatory medication while maintaining a tolerable level of activities. In addition, findings of shortened muscle bands forming nodularity may respond to dry needling.[28]

Avoidance of complete bed rest is preferred unless the condition is so severe that any activity is refused by the patient, and then bed rest should only occur for a few days with explanation of disuse atrophy and psychological deterioration. It is also suggested that the clinician reassure the patient that incurred discomfort from activity is expected and not harmful.

Finally, it is important to institute exercises early to diminish the duration of the acute phase and to begin a program to avoid recurrence. (Fear of recurrence is prominent in the patient's mind.) Exercise must be instituted to regain flexibility in all directions and to strengthen the stabilizing muscles of the trunk (transversus and quadratus lumborum). Exercises also have value in regaining flexibility and muscle tonus that are necessary for spinal stability. Exercises not only improve the mechanical stability of the low back but also permit resumption of normal activities of daily living.

Acute Low Back Pain Management

Appropriate management of acute low back pain is important to avoid chronicity, which is much more difficult to manage. The risk of chronicity is reduced by:[29]

- Paying attention to the psychological aspects of symptoms presentation,
- Avoiding unnecessary, excessive, or inappropriate investigation or treatment modalities,
- Avoiding inconsistent care,
- Giving advice on preventing recurrence (such as by sensible lifting and avoiding excessive loads),
- Avoiding prolonged bed rest during the acute phase as it causes disuse atrophy and psychological deterioration,
- Assuring the patient that "backache is not a serious disease and it should not cripple you unless you let it,"
- Explaining the difference between "hurt" and "harm,"
- Reassuring the patient about the future and the benign nature of the symptoms,
- Advising that analgesic drugs be taken on a regular basis and not on a pain contingent basis,
- Identifying the "red flags" to indicate the small number of patients who need referral for surgical intervention,
- Making necessary referrals for surgical intervention early when it can be more effective and accepted, and
- Managing distress and anger.

Exercises

Probably the most important modality of treating low back pain and impairment, whether acute, recurrent, chronic with radiculopathy or not, is exercise. Exercises regain flexibility in all directions: flexion, extension, lateral flexion, and rotation. Done with some resistance, exercises increase strength, tonus, and endurance of all of the stabilizing muscles, especially the trans versus and quadratus lumborum.[30,31] These two muscles are the most pertinent muscles to strengthen.

Strong abdominal muscles are vital in creating stability of the lumbar spine, which must be emphasized to the patient. Pelvic tilting exercises promote strength and tonus of these stabilizing muscles.

Teaching ergonomics is also important. *Ergonomics* indicates "how" the body must be used mechanically. How to bend, lift, push, pull, and lift overhead must be explained. However, it must be understood by the clinician and by the patient that all of the training and its repeated practice becomes unoperative when there is distraction or anger.

Recurrent Low Back Pain

Recurrence of low back pain is a fear that many patients experience. Recurrence occurs from several factors: poor conditioning from failure to participate in daily exercises; improper body mechanics resulting from depression or anger; or the task causing the pain has been excessive or greater than the intended effort managed. An example of the latter is the intent to lift a light object that proves to be heavier or vice versa.

Chronic low back pain occurs when the treatment for the acute or recurrent problem has failed to benefit the patient. For example, inappropriate exercises, inadequate preparation of the patient for the performance of the exercises, or an undiagnosed psychological condition in the patient are all examples of failed treatment.

Treatment for chronic pain requires a multidiscipled team including a physical therapist to implement the exercise program, a psychologist or psychiatrist, and a primary physician who has training in treating chronic pain and all of its modalities and medications.

CERVICAL SPINE

In daily clinical practice the complaint of pain in the neck, or from the neck, with impairment of activities of daily living is frequent. The major causes of these symptoms are trauma and arthritis.

Trauma

Trauma implies an external force having been applied to the cervical spine causing damage to tissues resulting in nociception and impaired function.[32] Trauma can be considered as an acute episode or as a prolonged stress such as ergonomic posture. The sequel of these forces produce resultant muscular contraction (spasm), which becomes a secondary impairment.

Emotional stress with resulting muscular tension is also a factor that causes impairment and pain from inflammation of the sensitive tissues of the cervical spine.

Ergonomic postural insult to the cervical spine can be exemplified in the current use of the computer in industry and the home where the head is held for long periods of time with infrequent breaks. The position of the head is determined by the angle of the computer screen and the distance and position of the operator. Also involved in this occupational stress is the intensity of the mental concentration of the operator, which causes prolonged muscular contraction with the head held in a position deviant to the center of gravity. The weight of the head is also an aggravating factor (Figure 2.17).

The history of this syndrome is neck pain, headache of an occipital site, limited range of motion as the facets become compacted, and radicular symptoms if and when the emerging nerve roots become compressed.

In evaluating the history and performing a physical examination to evaluate the pathomechanics of the impairment and the pain, it must be remembered that movement of the lower cervical spine is a conjoined movement with lateral flexion always associated with rotation and vice versa, and that these movements occur about the facet joints (Figure 2.18). Often rotation is limited to one side with pain upon reaching the end point of the motion.

To verify the site of neck pain and limitation, a physical examination of the neck is accomplished by having the patient actively move the head in all directions then repeating these motions passively.

Pain and impairment of the cervical spine has been postulated to occur from facet inflammation. Tenderness over a facet joint claimed to produce pain and limitation may be specifically confirmed by manually palpating each facet joint. Further confirmation may be achieved by injecting an analgesic agent into that joint. If the pain subsides, this procedure will also have a therapeutic effect. An x-ray, computed tomography (CT) scan, or MRI can document the exact tissue component and degree of the facet separation.

FIGURE 2.17

Computer Cervical Strain (1) The forward head posture needed to view the computer screen places the lower spine ahead of the center of gravity. (2) The head and upper cervical spine must extend (3), especially is bifocal glasses are needed. (4) Hyper-extension of the head irritates upper cervical units and may cause headaches. (5) The extended position causes compression of the facets and (6) posterior compression of the cervical thoracic unit may cause local pain.

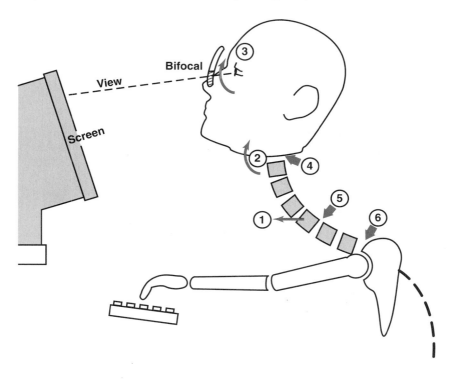

If there are neurological symptoms and findings implicating nerve root compression within the foramen, the compression and its specific site can be determined by performing the Spurling test and an appropriate neurological examination of the dermatomes and the myotomes of the upper extremity (Figure 2.19). Digital pressure by the examiner over the foramen also can elicit radiation into the dermatomal areas of the upper extremity.

In summary, the following tissue sites of the cervical spine as sites of nociception can be stated as:

■ the outer layers of the disk annulus,

■ the posterior longitudinal ligament,

FIGURE 2.18

Lateral Conjoined Cervical Movement The center figure illustrates the cervical spine from the front without lateral flexion or rotation. Bilaterally the foramen are equally open. With right lateral flexion, the foramen on the concave side close and those on the convex side open. Rotation is also shown. The right figure shows the upper cervical segment.

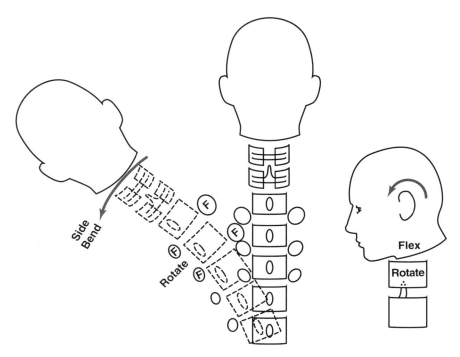

- the dural sheath of the nerve root,
- the dorsal root ganglion,
- the capsule of the facets,
- the erector spinae muscles, and
- the ligaments.

Degenerative Arthritis

Degenerative arthritis, considered a significant component of cervical spine impairment and pain, has been assumed to be a pathological diagnosis. It is essentially narrowing of the disk space with uncovertebral hypertrophy forming spurs at the vertebral levels and hypertrophic changes at the facet joints.

FIGURE 2.19

The Spurling Test A, With the head laterally flexed and rotated to the side of the symptoms, downward pressure on the head closes the foramen on the concave side and reproduce the symptoms in the upper extremity. B, Traction of the neck relieves the symptoms.

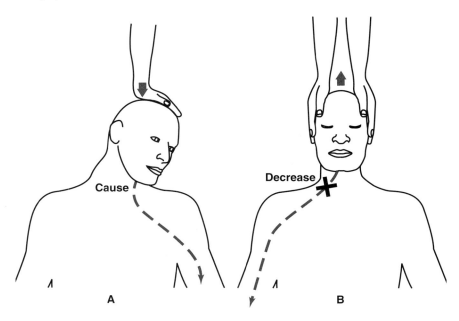

Disk degeneration is dehydration of the matrix with some damage to the annular fibers. These changes cause impairment of the hydrodynamics of the disk disrupting the stability of the functional units. The longitudinal ligaments following these hydrodynamic changes become lax and avulse from their attachments to the vertebrae. Blood invasion into the avulsed ligament ultimately calcifies and ossifies, becoming the spur (Figure 2.20).

These changes alter the freedom of motion with some discomfort upon reaching the end points of motion. The spurs encroach upon the foramen with narrowing that may impinge upon the contained nerve root, causing radicular signs and symptoms.

An article in *Lancet*[33] stated that the Bone and Joint section of WHO considered "research into osteoarthritis is at a critical watershed where many experts have abandoned the long held belief that it is a wear and tear disease . . . but is a disease of the entire joint." This is the concept of the proposed mechanism. The high metabolic

FIGURE **2.20**

Formation of a Spur A, Normal hydrodynamics of the disk (1) causing pressure against the posterior longitudinal ligament (PLL) (2). B, A decrease in disk hydrodynamics (3) with vascular invasion between the avulsed ligament (4) gradually becoming ossified (5) and forming a spur. D indicates disk; V, vertebra.

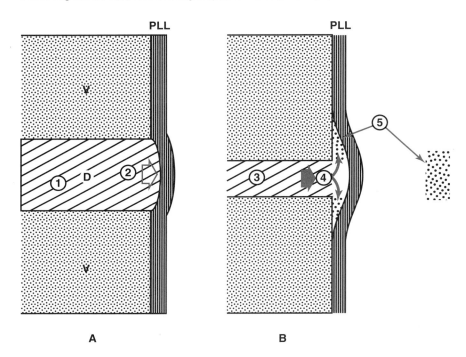

A   B

activity of thickened subchondral bone and the ligamentous laxity lead to the remodeling of the joint. "Osteoarthritis can be considered a complex disease with a factor of environmental risk and a strong genetic component."

In addition to these spurs and degenerated changes, peripheral nerve entrapment may result and the spinal canal may also narrow, causing compressive forces to the spinal cord and significant quadriplegia.

In addition to occurring at the lower cervical levels (C3-C7), pathology can also occur at the upper cervical levels (Figure 2.21). The neural components of the spinal canal here are the cord as well as the nerve roots, and trauma may injure one or both.

Any injury must be evaluated by performing a neurological examination for cord symptoms and signs as well as peripheral radicular

FIGURE 2.21

Cranio-Cervical Segments A, The occipital-atlas-axis units of the cervical spine. B, Only flexion (10 degrees) and extension (25 degrees) occurs at this level. The ligamentous stability of this segment is shown by the ligaments of the axis-atlas segments.

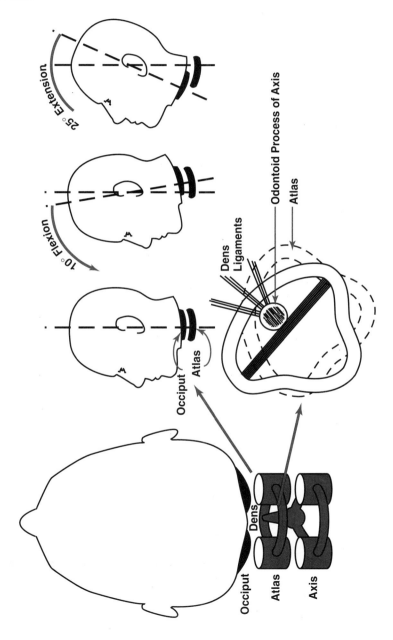

findings. Trauma to the upper cervical segments is often those of headaches. As concussion also occurs from a trauma to the upper cervical spine, this must be ruled out; however, headache may occur from insult to the C2-C3 segments entrapping the C2-C3 nerve roots that form the greater superior occipital nerve, which supplies the sensation to the posterior and lateral cranium.

The greater superior occipital nerve emerges at the base of the skull and can be palpated just medial to the mastoid process. Pressure there reproduces the symptoms and injection of an analgesic agent can eliminate the symptoms.

Whiplash-Associated Diseases

The so-called "whiplash syndrome" constitutes the most prevalent trauma to occupants of automobiles struck from the rear. This injury is particularly insidious with subtle pathology that often does not show up with radiological or other quantitative diagnostic techniques. Acute or chronic symptoms sometimes persist for years. The mechanics of whiplash are not well known and the correlation of tested animals and cadavers to humans is not exact. This was the summary of the Stapp Car Crash Conference held in Anaheim, California, on October 10-11, 1967. More recent conferences have not been more confirmatory.

The term *whiplash* was first introduced by an American orthopedist, H. E. Crowe, MD, in 1928, when he defined the effects upon the neck and upper trunk of a sudden acceleration-deceleration force. He considered the effect upon the neck as a "lash-like effect in which the head moved suddenly to produce a sprain in the neck."[34]

As there were, and are, many whiplash injuries sustained in vehicular injuries in Canada, the Quebec Task Force on Whiplash-associated Disorders (WAD) was created in 1995. This task force defined the effects of whiplash as "an acceleration-deceleration mechanism of energy transfer to the neck which may result from rear-end or side impact, predominantly in motor vehicle collisions but also from diving accidents, or from other mishaps."[35] The energy transfer may result in bony or soft tissue injuries (whiplash injuries), which in turn may lead to a wide variety of clinical manifestations.

The task force met in Vancouver, Canada, in 1999 to discuss their findings at the Whiplash Associated Disorders World Congress under the aegis of the Physical Medicine Research Foundation. At that meeting it was noted that "there is a lack of methodologic profound research on many aspects of WAD."[36]

The Quebec Task Force suggested the following classification as to the severity of a whiplash injury:

Grade 0: Whiplash exposure but no pain, no symptoms, no signs.

Grade 1: Delayed neck pain, minor stiffness, non-focal tenderness only, no physical signs.

Grade 2: Early onset neck pain, focal neck tenderness, spasm, stiffness, radiating symptoms.

Grade 3: Early onset neck pain, focal neck tenderness, spasm, stiffness, radiating, and signs of neurological deficit.

Grade 4: Neck complaint (Grade 2 or 3 above) and fracture dislocation.

The Ministry of Transport (Ontario, Canada) database stated that 65% of post-motor vehicle accidents were Grade 1 severity; 15%, Grades 3 and 4; and 20%, Grade 2.[35] Such grading exemplifies the ambiguity of defining what really is a "whiplash injury" as it uses vague terms such as "stiffness," "spasm," "focal neck tenderness," and "radiating symptoms."

The Quebec Task Force reviewed 10,000 abstracts selected from 294 scientific papers printed in medical journals and accepted only 62 as being meritorious. In his text, Arthur C. Croft, DC, cites 570 references but not all were reviewed for accuracy, pertinence, or confirmed with double blind study.[37,38]

Simulated impacts have been studied extensively and essentially confirmed that a low speed impact with minimal or no damage to the impacted vehicle can and does cause significant musculoskeletal injury to the driver's, or occupant's head and neck.[35,36] Speed of 5 to 7 miles per hour of the impacting vehicle have been shown to be detrimental and causative of injury. The answer is not yet confirmed but is evolving.

In a whiplash injury the pathomechanics are clear: the thoracic spine is elongated from the impact and the movement of the car and its seat. This straightened thoracic spine elevates the head and straightens the cervical spine. The translation forces then causes the vertebra to shear in a horizontal direction instead of its normal flexion extension (Figure 2.22). Impingement of the facets cause the major pain syndrome as well as does closure of the foramen upon the enclosed nerve roots.

In addition to mechanical compression of the nerve roots within the foramen, other factors play a role in acute trauma such as WAD.

FIGURE **2.22**

Translation Forces upon the Spinal Ligament A, Normal flexion where the vertebra flexes forward and in a downward direction (1), opening the foramen and gliding the facets forward. Extension (dotted lines) show the reverse, with the facets impinging upon each other (2). B, Translation forces (3) narrowing the disk space (4) and impinging the facets anteriorly (5).

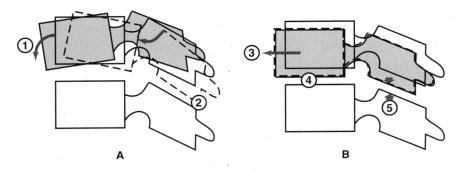

A   B

The nerve tissues within the canal are incompressible, but the cerebrospinal fluid within the foramen and the dura is altered.[39,40] During the rapid flexion-extension motion pressure gradients within the spinal column vary, causing variation of the spinal fluid with compression of the vein-plexi of the epidural space. These plexi do not have valves, allowing blood to flow in any direction and compression of the nerve roots to occur (Figure 2.23).

A translatory force upon the disk tissue can also cause annular tearing with posterior migration of the nucleus impinging on the posterior longitudinal ligament, which is pain sensitive. The uncovertebral joints protect the cord and the contents of the foramen to a degree, but may also be factors in causing damage to the disk, which occur more from rotatory factors (Figure 2.24).[32,41]

Diagnosis

The patient's statements are the only valid source of diagnosis, which admittedly, is subjective and from which is difficult to ascertain which anatomical tissues are the source of the complaints. Radiological studies, x-rays, CT scanning, and MRI are also nonspecific and when confused with aging changes, fail to objectify the bony and soft tissue changes. MRI studies of persons with no symptoms had abnormalities and increase with increasing age.

The history reveals the causative factors of the cervical pain and/or its radiation symptoms and findings. Passive and active movement

FIGURE 2.23

Spinal Fluid Course The spinal fluid (SF) fills the dural sac, which encloses the nerve root (NR), its dorsal root ganglion (DRG), and the spinal cord (SC). The veni-plexi (VP) that supply the spinal fluid are shown. V indicates the vertebra.

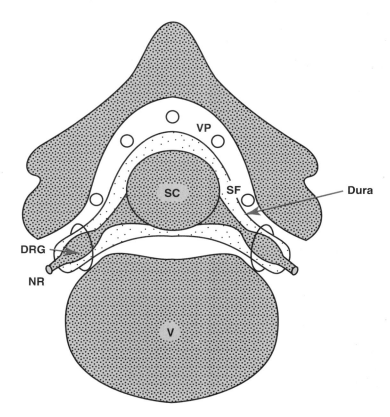

of the head and neck reveal the tissue site of the pain. As the facets are the most frequent site of pain and impairment there is tenderness over these joints and a specific level can be determined. Confirmation is afforded by x-ray studies, and if needed, an injection of an analgesic agent into the joint will determine whether that joint is the site of the symptoms. Relief of symptoms from the injection also may indicate a modality for treatment.

Treatment

If manual traction affords benefit, a trial of mechanical traction may be indicated and used as a home therapy program (Figure 2.25).

FIGURE **2.24**
Rotatory Injury to the Disk from the Uncovertebral Joints A, The presence of the uncoverteral process (UVP) and the horizontal tear in the annulus. B, Upon rotation and simultaneous lateral flexion, the inferior uncovertebral process becomes the axis of rotation about which the movement occurs, tearing the annular fibers.

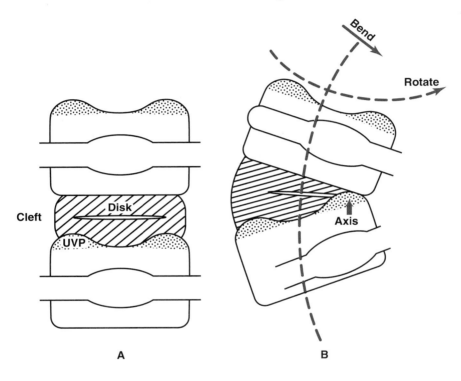

A   B

Exercises to strengthen the short flexors and the long extensors of the neck, which decrease the lordosis and increase stability, should be instituted (Figure 2.26). The prime movers of the neck are not stabilizing muscles and do not need attention (Figure 2.27).

Exercises to accomplish this stability include the deep short flexor muscle exercise (Figure 2.28), the isometric contraction of the short cervical muscles exercise (Figure 2.29), and the "flat neck" exercises (Figure 2.30). In addition, ergonomic training is dependent on discovering the positions of daily activities that initiate or aggravate the neck problems. These should be remedied as part of the treatment protocols.

FIGURE 2.25

Home Cervical Traction With a head halter and a pulley, the home cervical traction method is illustrated using tolerable weight (W) and assuring a 20-degree flexion.

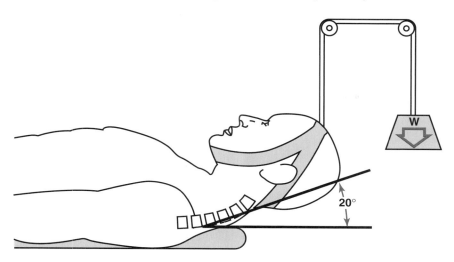

Cervicogenic Headache

The notion that headaches can occur from cervical problems and be relieved by treatment directed to the spine is widely recognized; however, it is rarely discussed in the literature and its patho-mechanics are not fully accepted or understood. In an article by Halderman,[42] a critical review of the literature, he concluded that "despite a growing body of literature . . . there remains considerable controversy and confusion concerning all aspects of this topic . . . the significance of radiological findings and advanced diagnostic testings is unclear . . . a clinician must be wary of enthusiastic and dogmatic claims concerning cervical diagnostic headaches."

THORACIC SPINE

Clinical Relevance

For centuries the dorsal kyphosis has been in the medical literature under the title of "posture."[1,3,5,6,43,44] "Traditionally a straight upright posture is associated with good health and vigor. Conversely a bent over posture is associated with poor health. Weak muscles,

FIGURE 2.26

Deep Muscles of the Neck The deep muscles of the neck are the semispinalis capitis (SC), obliquus capitis (OCI), rectus capitis minor and major (RCM), hyoid and suprahyoid muscles (H), rectus capitis anterior and lateralis (RC), and longissimus capitis (LC). These deep muscles are the stabilizing muscles of the neck.

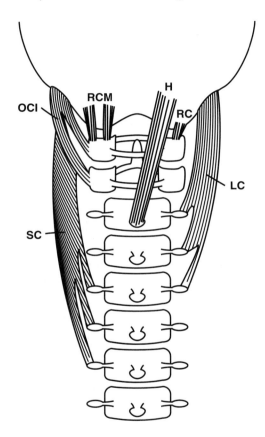

osteoporotic bones, deformed joints, and a variety of neurological conditions may, and often do, cause a bent posture."[1]

Excessive kyphosis may narrow the rib cage with respiratory difficulty, but most complications are related to the organs adjacent to the rib cage and the dorsal spine. Especially prominent as a complication are shoulder disorders. In a rounded back (dorsal kyphosis) the scapula rotates downward, placing the overhanging acromium at a lower level and causing impingement of the greater tuberosity on upper extremity abduction and forward flexion.[45,46]

FIGURE 2.27

Superficial Long Muscles of the Neck The long muscles of the neck are prime movers of the head and neck. They are the stenocleidomastoid (SCM), splenius capitis and cervicis (SCC), and scalene medius and anticus (SCL). ST indicates the sternum.

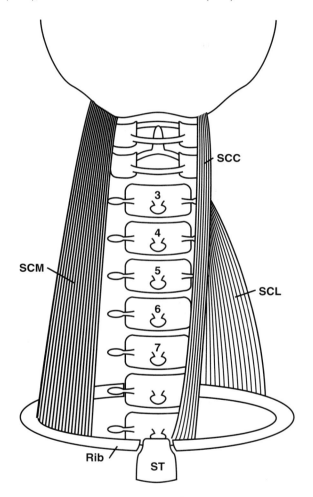

With a downward shoulder (scapula) rotation, the muscles of the scapula are also placed in stress and several muscular conditions evolve. The levator scapulae muscle and upper trapezius develop tension myositis and cause what is termed the *scapulocostal syndrome*. With excessive kyphosis the superincombent cervical spine undergoes compensatory lordosis and numerous painful syndromes occur.

FIGURE 2.28

Deep Short Flexor Muscle Exercise In the supine position (1) the cervical lordosis (dotted lines) is decreased as the patient forces the neck against the table. While holding that position (2) the patient lifts the head, but only to the extent of it being off the table (3).

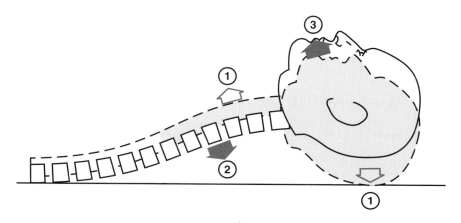

FIGURE 2.29

Isometric Contraction of the Short Cervical Muscles With the head held erect, the cervical lordosis is decreased. The patient presses against the forehead, which is resisted contracting the short neck flexors.

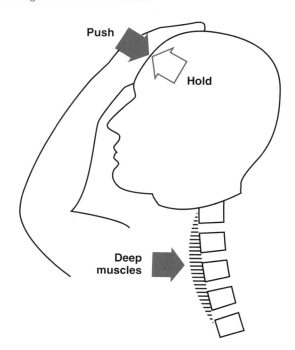

FIGURE 2.30

"Flat Neck" Exercises in the Erect Posture In the erect posture with the head against a wall, the neck is pressed against the wall (1). With a weighted sandbag on the head, the bag is pushed to contract the short neck flexors (2).

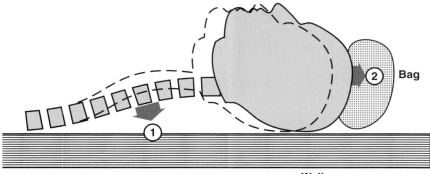

White and Panjabi[47] summarized that the clinical biomechanics of symptomatic kyphosis involve an equilibrium between the compressive forces borne by the anterior elements and the tensile forces borne by the posterior elements. They quote numerous statistics based on the Cobb angle measurement as varying between 20 degrees and 50 degrees, but define thoracic kyphosis with a posterior convexity measuring greater than 50 degrees.

Curves within several degrees of the 50-degree measurement and not associated with pain "may be difficult to define as abnormal."[47] The thoracic spine is subject to compression and flexion as a result of the center of gravity. There may be a decrease in the anterior width of the thoracic vertebrae causing a "wedging" with a segmental kyphosis that becomes deforming and painful. This is particularly true after trauma or in the presence of osteoporosis.

As the thoracic spine is a relatively inflexible structure, exercises, albeit often recommended, are usual ineffective.

SCOLIOSIS

Idiopathic scoliosis is a three-dimensional deformity of the spine with lateral curvature combined with vertebral rotation.[48] It is so termed as it is a pathological entity of unknown etiology. It was originally described by Hippocrates, but the term *scoliosis* was first used by Galen (AD 131-201) and *idiopathic scoliosis* was introduced in the middle of the nineteenth century by Bauer.[49]

Historically the cause initially was considered to be postural and poor nutrition, but over the decades there have been extensive studies as to etiology, pathomechanics, and etiological factors, but as yet, a definitive etiology has not been confirmed nor fully accepted. Numerous factors have been explored including melatonin abnormalities, genetics, collagen, neuromuscular, spinal musculature, platelet calmadulin, and thrombocyte abnormalities. Currently the diagnosis and treatment of scoliosis remains mechanical with bracing, casting, exercise, electrical stimulation, and surgical correction, but prevention remains aloof and all postulated causes remain unanswered.[50]

Genetic Factors

The role of genetic or hereditary factors is currently well accepted and documented. Harrington[51] studied women with scoliotic curves that exceed 15 degrees and a 27% prevalence of daughter-mother relationship. Studies of twins have shown that monozygous twins have a higher incidence by 73%, whereas dizygous twins had a concordant rate of 36%.[52-54] In spite of these studies there is no definite proof of any genetic mechanism;[48] although, "collectively studies characterize idiopathic scoliosis as a single-gene disorder that follows the simple patterns of Mendelian genetics."[50]

Pathomechanics of Idiopathic Scoliosis

As the anatomical abnormalities present the current problem to medical intervention, these factors remain predominant in clinical evaluation and intervention. The structural deformity is caused by a wedging of the vertebra and the intervetebral disks that is greater than the vertebra (Figure 2.31).

The intervertebral disks consist of collagen fibers within a matrix of proteoglycan. Pedrini et al[55] found a decrease in the glycosaminoglycan level in the disk nucleus pulposus with a concomitant rise in collagen levels. Whether this was causative or secondary to compressive forces upon the disk was debated, but it indicated some discogenic disease.[56]

Structural scoliosis has been produced by various surgical procedures: unilateral rib resection causing a thoracic rotoscoliosis, hemileminectomy, transection of posterior costotransversus ligaments,

FIGURE 2.31

Structural Changes in Spinal Segments in Scoliosis A, Normal alignment of the spine. B, The scoliotic spine with narrowing of the vertebral bodies (Vn) and narrowing of the disks (Dn) on the concave side. The dark arrows illustrate the compressive forces upon the disk. V indicates vertebra; D, disk.

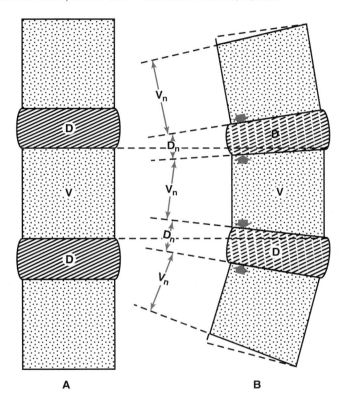

and fusion of transverse processes of thoracic vertebrae.[57] The resulting scoliosis of these procedures would be classified as acquired scoliosis and not idiopathic.

Growth Defects

As scoliosis may progress during spinal growth if the epiphyseal plates on the concave side receive abnormal pressure and no excessive pressure on the convex side, this may result in lateral scoliosis at those levels. Harrington[51] concluded that scoliosis has an extraosseous cause and the bone (vertebral and disk) changes are secondary.

Paravertebral Muscular Factors

The paravertebral muscles exert shearing and compressive forces upon the vertebral functional units (two adjacent vertebrae, their intervening disks, the facets posteriorly, and the ligaments) and can deform the unit.

Spencer and Eccles[58] described two types of muscle fibers in paravertebral muscles in patients with adolescent idiopathic scoliosis: Type 1 fibers, which are slow twitch; and Type 2, which are fast twitch. They found that Type 2 fibers were decreased in patients with adolescent idiopathic scoliosis, indicating that there was a muscle factor in this condition. Bylund et al[59] found normal distribution of Type 1 and Type 2 fibers on the convex side of the curve but a lower frequency on the concave side. This discrepancy indicates contraction, causing the bowing. However, increased electromyographic activity has been found in the muscles, but on the convex side of the curve, casting a doubt.[60]

Biopsy studies found a decrease in the muscles in patients with idiopathic scoliosis and a marked increase in calcium content, implying a generalized membrane defect.[61,62] These muscle abnormalities are likely to be secondary to the deformity rather than causative,[50] although they might indicate a defect in cell membranes.[63]

All of these experimental factors indicate why electrical stimulation of paraspinous muscles have failed to prevent or correct scoliosis but there are no studies in my search as to whether mechanical correction of a scoliosis alters the type and quantity of paraspinous muscles. A decrease in muscle spindles in paraspinous muscles has been found, which possibly could cause abnormal muscle contraction.

Melatonin and Serotonin

Thillard,[64] Dubousset et al,[65] and Dubousset and Machida[66] created scoliosis in chickens after they underwent a pinealectomy, creating the first experimental scoliosis with similar anatomical factors as humans. Machida produced similar scoliosis after pineal gland resection in rats.

The pineal gland primarily produces melatonin, which is an indole produced from tryptophan with serotonin as an intermediary. Serotonin may be involved in producing scoliosis in chickens but does not prevent development of scoliosis.[67] 5-hydroxytryptophan, a precursor of serotonin, appears to halt progression of scoliosis in pinealectomized chickens, but it is not effective in correcting an acquired scoliosos.

Bagnall et al[68] suggested that melatonin acted as a growth hormone, as an increase in scoliosis curvature was noted in patients undergoing growth-hormone therapy, but the pharmacological relationship between melatonin and growth hormone remains unclear.[69]

There is a diurnal variation in melatonin levels that appear important in the production of scoliosis as there is no evidence that patients with scoliosis have the inability to form melatonin nor do they have sleep difficulty or immune functional impairment, which is noted in a decrease of melatonin.

As the role of melatonin in the formation of scoliosis remains unclear, it can be concluded that melatonin plays a secondary role in idiopathic scoliosis and that the development of scoliosis does not occur merely from the absence of melatonin, but an alteration in the control of melatonin.[50]

Calmodulin

Increased activity in calmodulin has been noted in progressive scoliosis and can be considered a good predictor of potential progression.[70,71] Calmodulin is related to defects in platelets—their morphology and physiology—and may indicate a cell membrane defect.

Thus the following questions remain: "What is the relationship between calmodulin and melatonin in human idiopathic scoliosis?" "Does melatonin play a role in the creation of scoliotic deformity or in its progression?" "Are current findings secondary?" The answers to these questions may play a role in controlling the progression of idiopathic scoliosis once the condition is found to exist but at present, play no role in the management of the condition.

Connective Tissue

Collagen and elastic fibers are principal elements in the structures that support the vertebral column. Damage of disks and vertebral bodies causing scoliosis is noted on x-rays and MRIs and abnormal changes in glycosaminoglycans are evidence of connective tissue damage.

Neurological Mechanisms

Abnormal neurological mechanisms have been postulated for decades as a causative factor of scoliosis but to date, none has been confirmed. In studies, scoliosis developed in animals with central nervous system damage, especially on the convex side with damage found in the posterior horn and posterior gray matter.[72-74]

Yamada[75,76] postulated that any nervous system that disrupted the postural reflexes can cause scoliosis. Dysfunction of the vestibular system can cause scoliosis or, at least, was present in patients developing scoliosis,[77] but Yamada was unable to find any vestibular disorders.

Diagnosis

The presence of scoliosis is clinically discovered in routine examination of children in school evaluations or by pediatricians who do an examination for another concern. Parents may inadvertently discover the presence of scoliosis in seeing their child undressed.

The diagnosis is made by observing the child undressed and standing erect and viewed from behind. A plumb line applied from the base of the skull in the midline reveals any deviation of alignment. The child should then be made to flex as if attempting to touch the fingers to the toes. Any rotation is noted, which is the most important abnormality.

X-rays of the patient standing are then taken. The curves, if present, are measured and recorded. The Cobb method has been standard, although other methods have been proposed (Figure 2.32).[78,79] Ultimately a severe scoliosis may result that present cosmetic abnormality as well as potential pain.

Treatment

Today the curvatures are corrected and ultimately maintained by casting and/or bracing with dynamic braces that allow for gradual correction. Curves that progress to between 40 degrees and 50 degrees in skeletally immature patients progress at approximately 1 degree per year.[80] Exercises alone are not corrective but are valuable in maintaining balance upon closure of the epiphysis. They must be continued long after the braces are removed and especially in adults who have closed their epiphysis.

FIGURE 2.32

Cobb Measurement of Curvatures The lumbar curvature is measured by the Cobb method with the secondary curve attempting to return to the center of gravity (CG). The level of the iliac crests (IC) must be measured as they indicate a lumbar/pelvic ratio (LPR) and must be corrected. In this case the spine is left of the center of gravity, which is a detrimental factor.

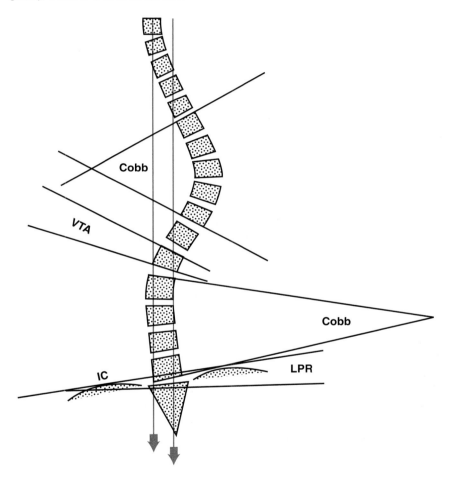

REFERENCES

1. Roaf R. *Posture*. London, England: Academic Press; 1977.

2. Nachemson A. Lumbar intradiscal pressure. In: Jayson MIV, ed. *The Lumbar Spine and Back Pain*. 2nd ed. Tunbridge Wells, England: Pitman Medical; 1980.

3. Phelps WM, Kiputh RJH, Goff CW. *The Diagnosis and Treatment of Postural Defects*. Springfield, Ill: CC Thomas; 1956.

4. Joseph J. *Man's Posture: Electomyographic Studies*. Springfield, Ill: CC Thomas; 1960.

5. Lowman CL, Young CH. *Postural Fitness*. Philadelphia, Pa: Lea & Febiger; 1960.

6. Lovett RW. *Lateral Curvature of the Spine and Round Shoulders*. Philadelphia, Pa: P Bakiston's Son & Co; 1907.

7. Thomas CL, ed. *Taber's Cyclopedic Medical Dictionary*. 16th ed. Philadelphia, Pa: FA Davis Co; 1989.

8. Nachemson A. The influence of spinal movements on the lumbar intradiscal pressure and on the tensile stresses in the annulus fibrosus. *Acta Orthop Scand*. 1963;33:183-207.

9. Nachemson A, Elfstrom G. Intravital pressure measurements in lumbar discs: a study of common movements, maneuvers and exercises. *Scand J Rehabil Med*. 1970;1:1-40.

10. Sato K, Kikuchi S, Yonezawa T. In vivo intradiscal pressure measurements in healthy individuals and in patients with ongoing back problems. *Spine*. 1999;24:2468-2474.

11. Andersson BJ, Ortengren R, Nahemson A, Elfstrom G. Lumbar disc pressure and myoelectric back muscle activity during sitting: I. Studies on an experimental chair. *Scand J Rehabil Med*. 1974;6:104-114.

12. Wilke HJ, Neef P, Caimi M, Hoogland T, Claes LE, et al. New in vitro measurements of pressures in the intervertebral disc in daily life. *Spine*. 1999;24:755-762.

13. Wilke HJ, Wolf S, Claes LE, et al. In vitro simulated muscle groups increase stability and intradiscal pressure at the lumbar spine. *J Bone Joint Surg*. 1997;79(suppl):17:1977.

14. Nachemson A. Lumbar intradiscal pressure. In: Jayson MIV, ed. *The Lumbar Spine and Back Pain*. 2nd ed. Tunbridge Wells, England: Pitman Medical; 1980.

15. Ghosh P. *The Biology of the Intervertebral Disc*. Vol 1. Boca Raton, Fla: CRC Press Inc; 1988.

16. Huskins DWL. Biomechanical properties of collagen. In: Weiss JB, Jayson MIV, eds. *Collagen in Health and Disease*. London, England: Churchill Livingstone; 1982.

17. Wiesel SW, ed. *The Back Letter*. Philadelphia, Pa: Lippincott Williams & Wilkins; May 2000;15.

18. Waddell G, Burton AK. *Occupational Health Guidelines for Management of Low Back Pain at Work-Evidence Review*. London, England: Faculty of Occupational Medicine; 2000.

19. Croft P, Macfarlane GJ, Papageorgiou AC, Thomas E, Silman AJ. Outcome of low back pain in general practice: a prospective study. *Br Med J*. 1998;316:1356–1359.

20. van Tulder MW, Assendelft WJ, Koes BW, Bouter LM. Methods guidelines for systemic reviews in the Cochrane Collaboration Back Review Group for Spinal Disorders. *Spine*. 1997;22:2323–2330.

21. Penfield W. Engrams in the human brain: mechanisms of memory. *Proc R Soc Med*. 1968;61:831–840.

22. Gunn CC. "Prespondylosis" and some pain syndromes following denervation supersensitivity. *Spine*. 1980;5:185–192.

23. Gunn CC. Radiculopathic pain: diagnosis and treatment of segmental irritation and sensitization. *J Musculoskeletal Pain*. 1997;5:119–123.

24. Cannon WB, Rosenbleuth A. *Supersensitivity of Denervated Structures*. New York, NY: The MacMillian Co; 1949.

25. Sicuteri F, Franchi G, Michelacci S. Biochemical mechanism of ischemic pain. *Adv Neurol*. 1974;4:39–43.

26. Klein L, Dawson MH, Heiple KG. Turnover of collagen in the adult rat after denervation. *J Bone Joint Surg Am*. 1977;59:1065–1067.

27. Nadler SF, Steiner DJ, Erasala GN, et al. Continuous low-level heat wrap therapy provides more efficacy than isoprofen and acetaminophen for low back pain. *Spine*. 2002;27:1012–1017.

28. Gunn CC, Milbrandt WE, Little AS, Mason KE. Dry needling of muscle motor points for chronic low back pain. *Spine*. 1980;5:279–291.

29. Main CJ, Williams AC. Musculoskeletal pain. *BMJ*. 2002;325:534–537.

30. Richardson C, Jull G, Hodges P, Hides J. *Therapeutic Exercise for Spinal Segmental Stabilization in Lower Back Pain*. Edinburgh, Scotland: Churchill Livingstone: 1999.

31. Cailliet R. *Low Back Disorders*. Philadelphia, Pa: Lippincott Williams & Wilkins; 2003.

32. Cailliet R. *Neck and Arm Pain*. 3rd ed. Philadelphia, Pa: FA Davis, Co; 1991.

33. Senior K. Osteoarthritis research: on the verge of a revolution? *Lancet*. 2000;355:208.

34. Nygren S, Cassidy JD. Whiplash: an important agenda for the future. In: Von Holst H, Nygren A, Thoird R, eds. *Transportation, Traffic Safety, and Health: The New Mobility*. Berlin, Germany: Springer Verlag; 1997.

35. Spitzer WO, Skovron ML, Salmi LR, et al. Scientific monograph of the Quebec Task Force on Whiplash-Associated Disorders: redefining "whiplash" and its management. *Spine*. 1995;20(8 Suppl):1-73.

36. Vernon H. Motor vehicle accident in Ontario: 1987-1994. *J Can Chirop Assoc*. 1998;2:171-173.

37. Croft AC. *Whiplash:1999, the Masters' Certification Program*. The Spine Research Institute of San Diego; 1998.

38. Croft AC. *Whiplash Injuries: The Cervical Acceleration/Deceleration Syndrome*. 2nd ed. Baltimore, Md: Lippincott Williams & Wilkins; 1995.

39. Breig A. *Adverse Mechanical Tension in the Central Nervous System*. Stockholm, Sweden: Almquist & Wilsell; 1978.

40. Svensson MY, Aldman B, Hansson HA, et al. Pressure effects in the spinal canal during whiplash extension motions: a possible cause of injury to the cervical ganglia. 1993 International ORCOBI Conference on the Biomechanics of Impacts. September 8-10, Einhoven, The Netherlands.

41. Taylor JR, Twomey LT. Acute injuries to cervical joints: an autopsy study of neck sprain *Spine*. 1993;18:1115-1122.

42. Halderman S, Dagenas S. Cervicogenic headaches. *Spine*. 2001;1:31-46.

43. Joseph J. *Man's Posture: Electromyographic Studies*. Philadelphia, Pa: CC Thomas; 1960.

44. Tribe DH. *Posture*. Australia; 1954.

45. Cailliet R. *Shoulder Pain*. 3rd ed. Philadelphia, Pa: FA Davis, Co; 1991.

46. Cailliet R. *Soft Tissue Pain and Disability*. 3rd ed. Philadelphia, Pa: FA Davis, Co; 1996.

47. White AA, Panjabi MM. *Clinical Biomechanics of the Spine*. 2nd ed. Philadelphia, Pa: Lippincott Williams & Wilkins; 1990.

48. Machida M. Cause of idiopathic scoliosis. *Spine*. 1999;24:2576-2583.

49. Goff CW. Louis Bauer: orthopedics extraordinary. *Clin Orthop*. 1956; 8:3-6.

50. Lowe TG, Edgar M, Margulies JY, et al. Etiology of idiopathic scoliosis: current trends in research. *J Bone Joint Surg*. 2000;82:1156-1168.

51. Harrington PR. The etiology of idiopathic scoliosis. *Clin Orthop*. 1977;126:17-25.

52. Esteve R. Idiopathic scoliosis in identical twins. *J Bone Joint Surg*. 1958;40:97-99.

53. Filho NA, Thompson MW. Genetic studies in scoliosis. In: Proceedings of the Scoliosis Research Society. *J Bone Joint Surg*. 1971;53:199.

54. Fisher RL, De George FV. A twin study of idiopathic scoliosis. *Clin Orthop*. 1967;55:117-126.

55. Pedrini VA, Ponseti IV, Dohrman SC. Glycosaminoglycans of intervertebral disc in idiopathic scoliosis. *J Lab Clin Med*. 1973;82:938-950.

56. Zaleske DJ, Ehrlich MG, Hall JE. Association of glycosaminoglycan depletion and degradative enzyme activity in scoliosis. *Clin Orthop*. 1980; 148:177–181.

57. Michelsson JE. The development of spinal deformity in experimental scoliosis. *Acta Orthop Scand*. 1965;81:1–19.

58. Spencer GS, Eccles MJ. Spinal muscle in scoliosis. Part 2. The proportion and size of type 1 and type 2 skeletal muscle fibres measured using a computer-controlled microscope. *J Neurol Sci*. 1976;30:143–154.

59. Bylund P, Jansson E, Dahlberg E, Ericksson E. Muscle fiber types in thoracic erector spinae muscles. Fiber types in idiopathic and other forms of scoliosis. *Clin Orthop*. 1987;214:222–228.

60. Reuber M, Schultz A, McNeill T, Spencer D. Trunk muscle myoelectric activities in idiopathic scoliois. *Spine*. 1983;8:447–456.

61. Ford DM, Bagnall KM, Clements CA, McFadden KD. Muscle spindles in the paraspinal musculature of patients with adolescent idiopathic scoliosis. *Spine*. 1988;13:461–465.

62. Yarom R, Robin GC. Studies on spinal and peripheral muscles from patients with scoliosis. *Spine*. 1979; 4:12–21.

63. Riddle HV, Roaf R. Muscle imbalance in the causations of scoliosis. *Lancet*. 1975;1:1245–1247.

64. Thillard MJ. Deformations de la colonne vertebrale consecutives a l'epiphysectomie chez le pussin. *Extrat des comptes Rendus de l'Association des Anatomistes*. 1959;751–758.

65. Dubousset J, Queneau P, Thillard MJ. Experimental scoliosis induced by pineal and diencephalic lesions in young chickens: its relation with clinical findings. *Orthop Trans*. 1983;7:7.

66. Dubousset J, Machida M. Melatonin: a possible role in the pathogenesis of human idiopathic scoliosis. In: Proceedings of Tenth International Philip Zorab Symposium on Scoliosis. Oxford, England: Oxford University Press; 1998.

67. Evans SC, Edgar MA. Hall-Craggs MA, Powell MP, Taylor BA, Noordeen HH. MRI of idiopathic juvenile scoliosis. A prospective study. *J Bone Joint Surg Br*. 1996;78:314–317.

68. Bagnall KM, Raso VJ, Hill DL, et al. Melatonin levels in idiopathic scoliosis. Diurnal and nocturnal serum melatonin levels in girls with adolescent idiopathic scoliosis. *Spine*. 1996;21:1974–1978.

69. Kawabata H, Ono K, Seguchi Y, Tanaka M. Idiopathic scoliosis and growth: a biomechanical consideration. *Nippon Seikeigeka Gakkai Zasshi*. 1988;62:161–170.

70. Kindsfater K, Lowe T, Lawellin D, Weinstein D, Akmakjian J. Levels of platelet calmodulin for the prediction of progression and severity of adolescent idiopathic scoliosis. *J Bone Joint Surg*. 1994;76:1186–1192.

71. Cohen DS, Solomons CS, Lowe TG. Altered platelet calmodulin activity in idiopathic scoliosis. *Orthop Trans.* 1985;9:106.

72. Alexander MA, Bunnch WH, Ebbersson SO. Can experimental dorsal rhizotomy produce scoliosis? *J Bone Joint Surg.* 1950;32:396-401.

73. Barrios C, Tunon MT, Salis JA, Beguiristain JL, Canadell J. Scoliosis induced by medullary damage: an experimental study in rabbits. *Spine.* 1987;12:433-439.

74. Barrios C, Arrotegui JI. Experimental kyphoscoliosis induced in rats by selective brain stem damage. *Int Orthop.* 1992;16:146-151.

75. Yamada K, Ikata T, Yamamoto H, Nakagawa Y, Tenaka H. Equilibrium function in scoliosis and active plaster jacket or the treatment. *Tokushima J Exp Med.* 1969;16:1-7.

76. Yamada K, Yamamoto H, Nakagawa Y, Tezuka A, Tamura T, Kawata S. Etiology of idiopathic scoliosis. *Clin Orthop.* 1984;184:50-57.

77. Sahlstrand T, Petruson B, Nachemson A. An electronystagmographic study of the vestibular function in patients with idiopathic scoliosis. 11th Annual Meeting of the Scoliosis Research Society. 1976; Ottowa, Ontario.

78. Harrison DE, Harrison DD, Cailliet R, Troyanovich SJ, Janik TJ, Holland B. Cobb method or Harrison posterior tangent method: which to choose for lateral cervical radiographic analysis. *Spine.* 2000;25:2072-2078.

79. Harrison DE, Harrison DD, Cailliet R, Janik TJ, Holland B. Radiographic analysis of lumbar lordosis: centroid, Cobb, TRALL, and Harrison posterior tangent methods. *Spine.* 2001;26:E235-E242.

80. Weinstein SL, Dolan LA, Spratt KF, Peterson KK, Spoonamore MJ, Ponseti IV. Health and function of patients with untreated idiopathic scoliosis: a 50-year natural history study. *JAMA.* 2003;289:559-567.

Shoulder Girdle

Pain and impairment of the shoulder is a prevalent condition that confronts all ages and both sexes. It would be better for the orthopedic profession to consider the condition as "shoulder girdle," because in everyday clinical practice, the term *shoulder* usually applies to only the glenohumeral joint and its immediate associated tissues. Although this joint predominates as the site of greatest impairment, other girdle joints also can be involved.

The function of the shoulder girdle is to place the hand into a functional position to permit manipulative activities. To do this implies that there are complex neuromuscular actions of numerous joints and muscles (Figures 3.1, 3.2).

In the patient with an impaired shoulder girdle, the presenting findings are pain and impairment of the arm motion at the gleno-humeral joint. The patient cannot place the hand in a functional position without pain and limitation of motion. Limited motion at the glenohumeral joint prevents forward flexion, abduction, external rotation, and overhead elevation.

GLENOHUMERAL JOINT PAIN

Clinically, a condition of "shoulder pain and impairment" implies tendinitis, rotator cuff disease, partial and/or complete tears of the rotator cuff, and even calcific tendinitis.

Functional Anatomy

To understand this impairment, the normal functional anatomy of the glenohumeral joint must be understood. The glenohumeral joint is composed of the glenoid fossa, which is at the lateral tip of the scapula and at the head of the humerus. The glenoid fossa is ovoid and shallow and is made deeper with the formation of the glenoid

FIGURE 3.1

Complex Neuromuscular Trajectory of Upper Extremity In trajectory phase of upper extremity, with hand and fingers in their functional position, scapular muscles—upper trapezius (UT), middle trapezius (MT), lower trapezius (LT), and anterior serratus (SA)—sustain scapula (S) with isometric contraction to support upper extremity (short arrows). Weight on upper extremity depends on distance of object from scapula. All neuromuscular aspects are determined by spindle system (Sp) and Golgi apparatus (Go) "reporting" to spinal cord (SC), with resultant afferent impulses causing appropriate muscular (M) contraction.

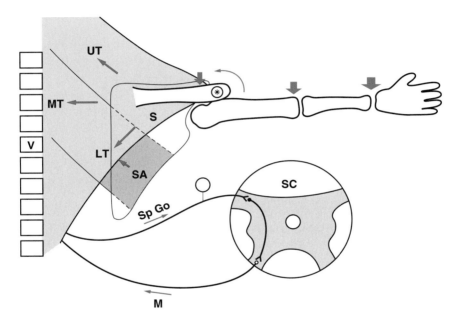

labrum. The glenohumeral joint is surrounded by the muscles of the joint in all aspects except the inferior border, which is enclosed merely by the capsule (Figure 3.3). The glenohumeral joint is a typical incongruous joint in that the opposing surfaces are asymmetrical (Figure 3.4).

The glenohumeral joint exemplifies *congruency*, which is an engineering term initially defined by MacConnaill.[1] The incongruity is that the convexity of the humeral head and the concavity markedly differ.

In the dependent position of the arm, the head of the humerus is held within the glenoid fossa by the supraspinous muscle, as the capsule is not strong enough to support the upper extremity. The

FIGURE 3.2

Planes of Arm Movement Planes of arm movement indicate direction of movement from body. All planes are related to coronal and sagittal planes.

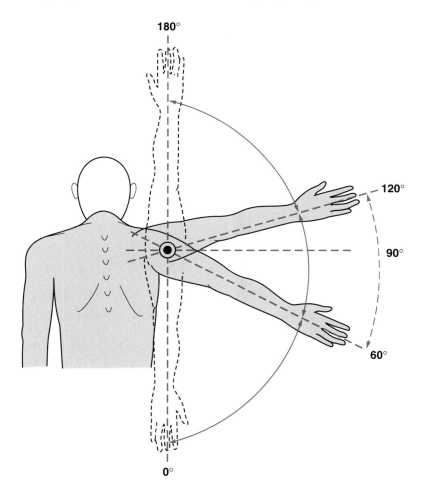

supraspinous muscle is in a sustained contraction, dictated by the spindle system (Figure 3.5).

As the arm moves to place the hand in a functional position, the head of the humerus glides downward or forward within the glenoid fossa as the supraspinous muscle contracts. As the humerus abducts (or forward flexes) at 90 degrees of abduction, the humerus

FIGURE 3.3

Muscles Forming Glenohumeral Joint Glenoid fossa (GF) is enclosed by supraspinous (SS), infraspinous (IS), teres minor (TM), subscapular (SSc), and latissimus dorsi (LD) muscles. Biceps tendon (BT) lies at superior aspect, and pectoral muscle (PM) lies anteriorly. GL indicates glenoid labrum.

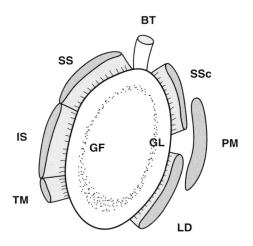

FIGURE 3.4

Congruity of a Joint A, Congruous joint with both surfaces (a, b, c, d) of equal distances. Axis of rotation (A) remains central during rotation, and muscles (M) act about this axis. C indicates capsule. B, Incongruous joint with 2 adjacent surfaces (h, e, f, g) that are unequal. As the head of the humerus glides rather than rotates, and axis (A) is no longer fixed. Capsule (C_1) also varies in its length.

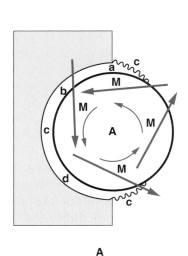

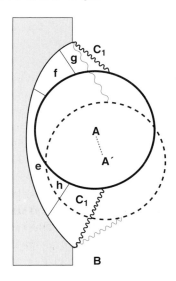

A

B

FIGURE 3.5

Support of Dependent Arm Supraspinous muscle (SS) isometrically contracts, by its attachment to greater tuberosity (GT) of humerus (H) and angulation of glenoid fossa (G), to prevent downward dislocation of humerus (x-x to x-y). CO indicates coracoid; AC, acromion; and IS, subscapular muscle, which is also part of conjoined tendon.

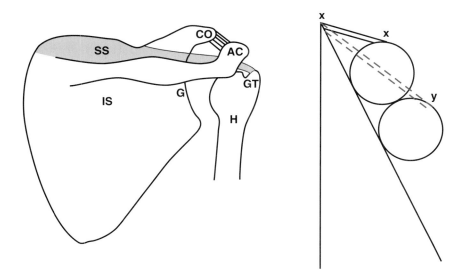

impinges on the acromion and/or the coracoacromial ligament (Figure 3.6).

As the humerus moves within the glenoid fossa, the scapula at first remains static while the humerus abducts and flexes to 90 degrees. Then the scapula performs what is called the *scapulohumeral rhythm,* in which the scapula rotates outward to move the overhanging acromion and coracohumeral ligament upward and away from the ascending humerus (Figure 3.7).

What causes tendinitis or rotator cuff tears is faulty abduction with inappropriate rotation. This impinges the rotator cuff on the acromion and the coracoacromial ligament (Figure 3.8). As the conjoined tendon becomes inflamed from compression and friction, it prevents movement of the tendon, thus impairing movement of the humerus through the first phase of the rhythm. The scapula begins its movement sooner and more completely, while the humerus becomes "fixed" with the glenoid fossa. The patient exhibits the "shrugging mechanism," which is characteristic of rotator cuff impairment (Figure 3.9).

FIGURE 3.6

Impingement of Greater Tuberosity on Coracoacromial Ligament and Acromion
A, In neutral rotation the greater tuberosity (GT) impinges upon the overhanging
acromion (AC). B, With the humerus externally rotated (ER), abduction is permitted
to 120 degrees. C, With the humerus internally rotated (IR), impingement occurs at
60 degrees.

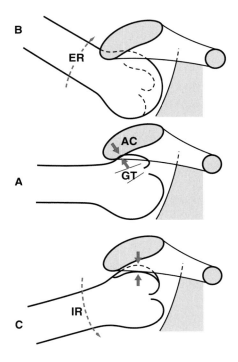

Because the supraspinous muscle is also an external rotator
(Figure 3.10), external rotation, both active and passive, is also limited and painful. The biceps tendon passively assists in the abduction
of the arm (Figure 3.11) and explains why biceps tendinitis often
accompanies rotator cuff inflammation.

All of the tissues coexist within the suprahumeral space and are
contiguous. Inflammation of one inflames the adjacent tissue, further
restricting movement, causing pain, and leading to potential "frozen
shoulder," or adhesive capsulitis (Figure 3.12).

FIGURE 3.7

Scapulohumeral Rhythm A, Dependent arm with scapula (S) and humerus (H) essentially parallel. AC indicates overhanging acromion. B, Humerus (H) abducting to 90 degrees, where it impinges on acromion. To avoid impingement, scapula (S) begins gradual rotation: 1 degree for every 2 degrees of humerus abduction-flexion, which is known as *2-1 scapulohumeral rhythm.* C, For overhead elevation of humerus (H, 180 degrees), scapula (S) has fully rotated. There has been rotation of humerus during this rhythm, as shown in Figure 3.6.

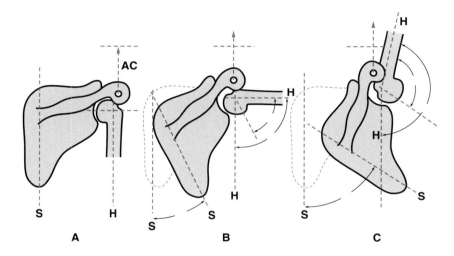

The head of the humerus is maintained within the glenoid fossa by the combined action of the rotator cuff and the capsule. However, excessive force causing the head to be forced downward within the glenoid fossa can dislocate the head through the area that has only capsule and no muscles (Figure 3.13).

As initially stated, the term *shoulder girdle* is more appropriate than merely "the shoulder," which often indicates the glenohumeral and suprahumeral joints. There are numerous other joints in the girdle, of which any or all may cause impairment and pain (Figure 3.14).

Diganosis

The clinical findings, history, and examination reveal the cause of the impairment and pain. Radiologic studies include x-ray films, which

FIGURE 3.8

Conjoined Tendon In a conjoined tendon, 4 tendons—supraspinous, infraspinous, subscapular, and teres minor—merge to attach to greater tuberosity of humerus (H). Biceps tendon passes through a hiatus. Acromiocoracoid ligament from acromion (AC) to coracoid is shown.

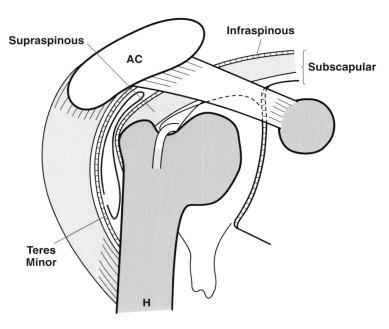

show only the bony structures and their relationship, whereas computed tomography (CT) scans and magnetic resonance imaging (MRI) studies reveal the soft tissue involved.

Treatment

The first approach in treating impairment of the glenohumeral joint is to decrease the inflammation of the conjoined tendon. Local application of ice is advisable periodically. Oral steroids are of value, and steroids can also be injected via a suprahumeral approach.

Movement to prevent adhesion of the inflamed tissues must be initiated immediately and is done with active-passive exercise. This paradox (active-passive) is exemplified by the Codman pendular

FIGURE 3.9

Shrugging Mechanism As the arm attempts to abduct movement of humerus at glenohumeral joint, it is impaired and scapula rotates excessively, causing arm to "shrug."

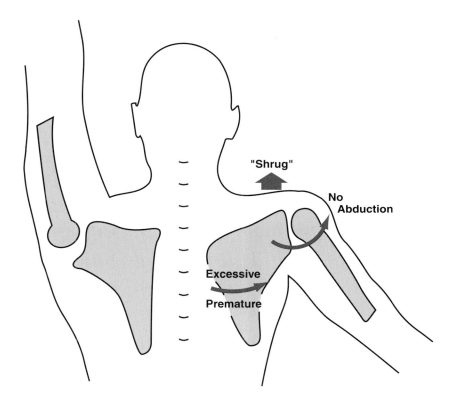

exercise, in which the pendular arm is actively moved in circumduction without implementation of the shoulder muscles (Figure 3.15).

As soon as tolerated, usually in 3 to 4 days, active exercises are initiated to ensure full range of motion and to increase the strength of the shoulder girdle muscles, especially the rotator cuff muscles (Figure 3.16). Overhead exercises can be performed with an overhead pulley using the other arm for the active phase.

FIGURE 3.10

External Rotation by Supraspinous Muscle Supraspinous muscle externally rotates (EXT) humerus (H), whereas subscapularis muscle internally rotates (INT) humerus. BT indicates biceps tendon.

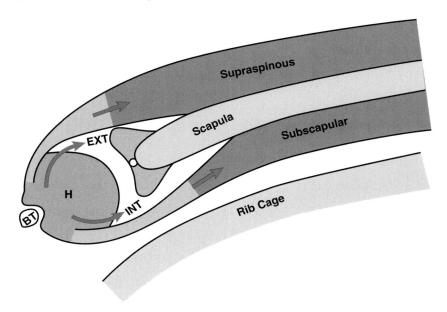

ACROMIOCLAVICULAR (AC) JOINT PAIN

History

Injury to the acromioclavicular (AC) joint usually results from direct trauma. The joint is a synarthrodial joint and not a synovial joint, and both ends are held together with fibrous and collagen fibers that permit merely rotation and little other motion.

The history designates the trauma, the site of pain, and which motions are painfully limiting. The examination may show evidence of inflammation, but usually only tenderness is noted. Crepitation may be heard and is reported by the patient to be painful. The movement that is most limited is elevation and circumduction of the shoulder girdle.

FIGURE 3.11

Biceps Mechanism Long head of biceps (B), which attaches to supraglenoid tubercle of scapula (GF), presses down on humeral head (H) as it abducts. Short head (SH) of biceps originates from coracoid process (C).

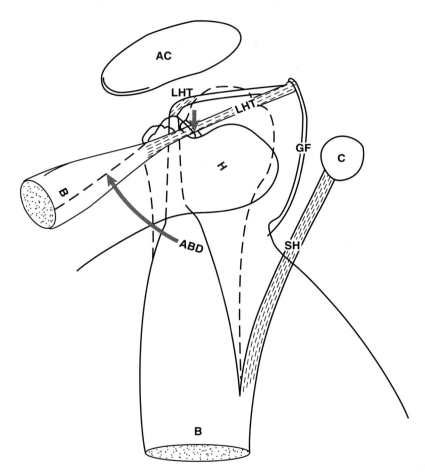

Diagnosis

Dislocation of the AC joint visually shows a deformity called *shoulder pointer*. In this deformity, the scapula falls away from the clavicle and the end of the clavicle is more prominent. This is noted when the undressed patient is viewed from the front where the scapula

FIGURE 3.12

Contiguous Synovial Tissues As all of the tissues contained within the suprahumeral space are contiguous and share adjacent synovial lining, when one becomes inflamed they become inherent. DM indicates to deltoid muscle; AC, acromion; CT, conjoined tendon; GT, greater tuberosity; BT, biceps tendon; H, head of humerus; GF, glenoid fossa; SDB, subdeltoid bursa, which shares lining of inferior deltoid and outer layer of conjoined tendon; and GHC, glenohumeral capsule.

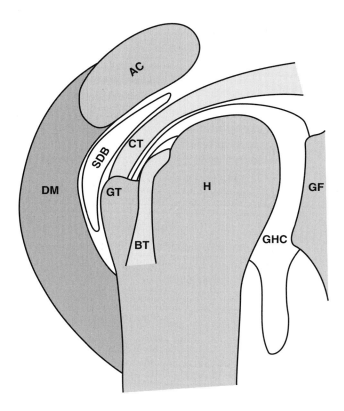

falls away from the clavicle and the acromium lies below and in front of the clavicle. Clinically there is tenderness over the palpable site of dislocation and when the clavicle is palpated from the sterno-clavicular joint distally to the acromium, there is a cleft noted that is not noted on the opposite side. Elevation, depression, and circum-duction of the shoulder girdle elicits painful crepitation that can be heard and felt.

FIGURE 3.13

Dislocation Site of Humeral Head Humeral head (HH) can dislocate from glenoid fossa (GF) inferiorly (arrows) where there is only capsule and no muscles. Among the muscles, SS indicates supraspinous; IS, infraspinous; TM, teres minor; SSc, sub-scapular; L, latissimus dorsi; and PM, greater pectoral. GL indicates glenoid labrum.

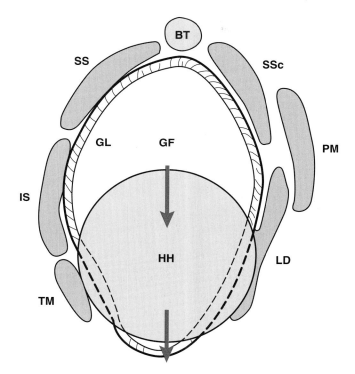

Injection of an analgesic agent such as lidocaine relieves the pain, which is diagnostic and therapeutic.

Treatment

Treatment involves the local application of ice and support of the arm with a sling that elevates the elbow upward toward the clavicle and depresses the upper trapezius, which approximates the AC joint. This immobilization must be applied for as long as three weeks. Injection of an analgesic with a steroid into the joint spaces decreases the pain. Surgical intervention is debatable, as it is not usually beneficial.

FIGURE 3.14

Joints of Shoulder Girdle These joints form shoulder girdle complex: (1) glenohumeral, (2) suprahumeral, (3) acromioclavicular, (4) scapulocostal, (5) sternoclavicular, (6) sternocostal, and (7) costovertebral.

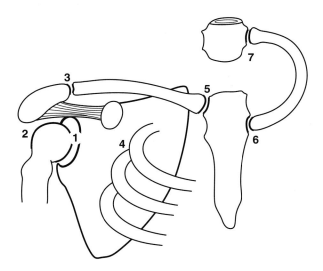

STERNOCLAVICULAR JOINT PAIN

History

Injury to the sternoclavicular joint is infrequent and usually occurs from direct trauma to the joint or acute depression of the shoulder girdle. When injury to the sternoclavicular joint occurs, pain is often accompanied by acromioclavicular pathology and thus may be lost in the diagnosis.

Diagnosis

After trauma, the patient usually notes pain and tenderness over the sternoclavicular joint that is aggravated by circumduction of the shoulder girdle. A deformity may be noted when compared to the opposite side.

Treatment

Benefit from local injection of a lidocaine solution into the joint is confirmatory and possibly therapeutic.

FIGURE 3.15

Codman Pendular Exercises With the person bent over, inflamed arm becomes dependent and the person makes circumduction motion by moving the total body. Arm moves passively, and body moves actively. No weight is used, as that would initiate active shoulder muscles to react, which would make them active.

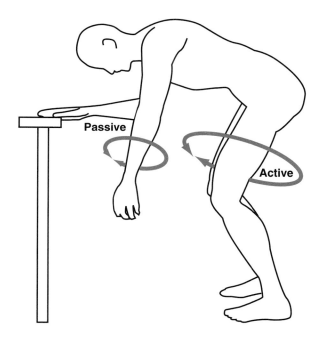

FIGURE 3.16

Active Shoulder Exercises Using elastic band, arm performs external rotation exercises.

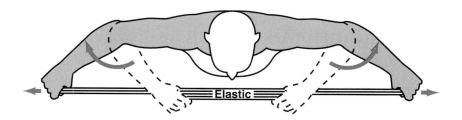

SCAPULOCOSTAL JOINT PAIN

History

The scapulocostal joint is a joint between the inferior aspect of the scapula and the thoracic chest wall. The scapula moves in conjunction with the shoulder girdle in scapulohumeral rhythm. As the scapula supports the entire upper extremity, it relies upon the scapular muscles, which are in a state of tonus in any erect position of the body. If there is a postural abnormality from prolonged ergonomic activities, the muscles of the scapula are strained and become the site of nociception.

Diagnosis

The patient may complain of pain in the scapulocostal area with pain and tenderness located in the superior medial aspect of the scapula, causing a diagnostic condition called *scapulocostal syndrome*. This condition frequently occurs due to prolonged dorsal kyphotic posture, or "round back." Scapulocostal syndrome may also be termed "computer musculoskeletal shoulder pain," because it is noted as a result of the pronged bent-over posture of the person spending hours at the computer.

The findings are tenderness at the site of insertion of the levator scapular muscle into the superior-medial border of the scapula. Pain is aggravated by this prolonged posture and may be accentuated by elevation and adduction of the scapula.

Treatment

Relief as well as diagnosis verification is afforded by an injection of an anesthetic agent with or without steroid into the trigger area.

THORACIC OUTLET SYNDROME

History

Although there are controversial opinions regarding the diagnoses of thoracic outlet syndrome, there are sufficient numbers of patients with the complaint to justify its being discussed and the anatomical structures of the outlet clarified. The *outlet* consists of the space

Thoracic Outlet Anterior scalene muscle (A) originates from lateral process of cervical vertebrae (CV, ie, C2 through C7) and descends to attach to the first rib. Middle scalene muscle (M) has similar origin but attaches more laterally to first rib, forming opening through which brachial plexus (BP, N) and subclavian artery (SCA) pass.

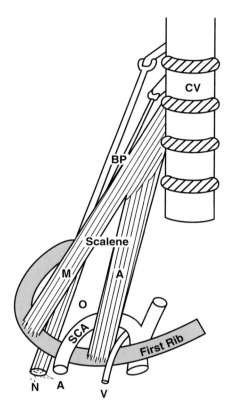

between the first rib and the scalene muscles; through those muscles pass the brachial plexus and the subclavian artery and vein as they descend as a neurovascular bundle between the first rib and the clavicle (Figure 3.17).

Diagnosis

Patients with this syndrome suffer paresthesia (numbness and tingling) of the hand with obliteration of the pulse at the wrist.

The neurologic symptoms and findings are usually of the lower trunk of the brachial plexus in the C8-T1 dermatomic and myotomic regions.

Symptoms can be reproduced or aggravated by activities that close the thoracic outlet, such as repeated overhead activities or carrying heavy objects. Clinically, symptoms are reproduced by performing the Adson test. This is done by elevation and posterior flexion of the symptomatic arm, having the patient's head extended and turned to the afflicted side, and having the patient inhale deeply and hold his or her breath. The pulse on the afflicted side diminishes or disappears, and the symptoms are reproduced.

No radiologic findings are diagnostic unless the patient has a cervical rib, which is considered a factor.

Treatment

Management of thoracic outlet syndrome is preferably conservative before surgical intervention is considered. Conservative measures include improving the posture, modifying the ergonomics of daily work, and strengthening the scapular muscles. Surgical intervention includes resection of a cervical rib and resection of the scalene muscles.

SHOULDER-HAND-FINGER SYNDROME

Any patient whose shoulder is painful and has limited motion, regardless of the cause, and who has a swollen hand must be considered for a diagnosis of shoulder-hand-finger syndrome.

History

This syndrome currently is considered to be a component of reflex sympathetic dystrophy and is termed complex regional pain syndrome (CRPS). However, shoulder-hand-finger syndrome can occur from mechanical factors without any sympathetic nervous system involvement, making its relationship to CRPS unclear.

The classic signs of CRPS are being generally defined, recognized, and researched. Shoulder-hand-finger syndrome, however, has been recognized much longer and remains a disabling syndrome.[2]

Diagnosis

The shoulder-hand-finger syndrome may occur after any incident that painfully impairs shoulder motion, such as tendinitis, rotator cuff injury, and frozen shoulder subluxation, as well as from a compound cerebral vascular accident. Shoulder-hand-finger syndrome may occur within the first few months after a stroke in approximately 12% of patients. Initially a painful swollen hand is noted after occurrence of shoulder pain with limited motion.[3,4] This syndrome occurring after a stroke usually has impairment of the hand due to the stroke present, which makes up the hand component of the syndrome.

In the patient who has suffered a complete stroke, the involved shoulder initially may be frail (no muscle tone), causing the arm to be totally dependent and unable to be elevated or abducted above the level of the heart. Once the flailing arm develops spasticity, the shoulder cannot function or allow elevation, abduction, or external rotation. The arm then becomes dependent but from a different shoulder problem, this time with loss of scapulohumeral rhythm.

After several months, the loss of motion in the shoulder and the muscular contraction impair the upper "pump," which propels the fluid within the arm and hand via arterial capillary action. The hand muscles within the forearm and the intrinsic finger muscles, which also propel the tissue fluids cardiac-wise through venous and lymphatic vessels, are defective and fluid accumulates in the hand (edema).

These "pumps" are the shoulder musculature, forearm musculature, and hand musculature. The "pumps" propel the circulation—venous and lymph—back to the heart and lungs after the blood has been moved to the upper extremity by cardiac contraction and compressive forces of the upper extremity "pumps" (Figure 3.18).

Elevation of the arm above heart level assists by gravity to return the venous and lymph flow from the extremity to the circulation. It is apparent that elevation of the arm above heart level must occur to facilitate the removal of fluid in the upper extremity, and this is impaired by the inability of the arm to abduct and elevate overhead. The hand also assists in pumping the tissue fluids from the arm but alone is not sufficiently strong enough to eliminate fluid against gravity with a dependent arm.

Persistent edema in the hand causes functional impairment, which may become chronic with total loss of function. Initially the

FIGURE 3.18

"Pumps" of Upper Extremity "Pumps" that occur from muscular contraction and joint movements of upper extremity are shoulder (S), forearm and hand (H), and fingers (F). Efficient blood flow to arm involves arterial blood supply (A) with efferent return flow via veins (V) and lymphatic vessels (L). Elevation of arm above heart level assists return flow from arm.

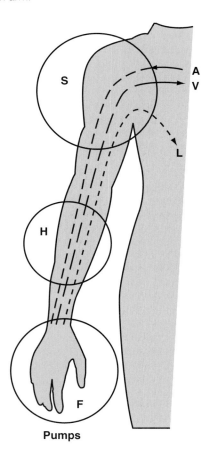

Pumps

edema is noted on the dorsum of the hand, where most of the venous and lymphatic vessels are located, with the arterial supply of the hand being mostly located on the volar palmar area. At first, the edema of the hand is noted in the skin on the dorsum of the fingers, with the skin becoming smooth and devoid of wrinkles. This edema is first noted at the metacarpophalangeal joints. The skin becomes pale, and pitting can be elicited. Flexion of the hand gradually

FIGURE 3.19

Metacarpophalangeal Flexion and Effects of Edema Metacarpal and proximal phalangeal flexion (F) and extension (E) occur about an ovoid curvature with initial downward gliding, then rotation around curvature of inferior surface (dashed curve). Collateral ligaments (CL) are relaxed during extension but become taut at full flexion. Edema gets between extensor tendon and under collateral ligaments, causing ligaments to become taut and restricting flexion. Edema under extensor tendon also limits flexion.

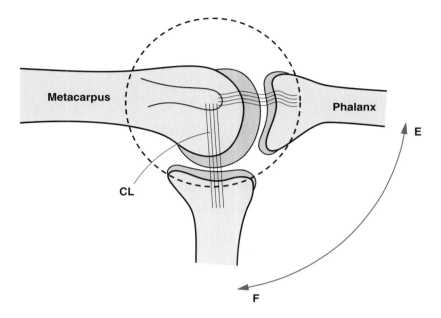

diminishes until a full fist cannot be made. If this persists or progresses, the muscles atrophy and contracture of all the periarticular joints occurs. The hand becomes dystrophic and useless.

The mechanism of this hand component is explainable. Normally the metacarpophalangeal joint flexes in a specific manner due to the curvature of the head of the metacarpus. This surface is rhomboid (Figure 3.19). For the proximal phalanx to flex, it must descend parallel to the superior flat surface of the head of the metacarpus until the rotation occurs that permits the joint to flex.

Edema that forms under the extensor tendon and under the collateral ligaments restricts flexion. If edema is permitted to remain, it undergoes fibrous reaction with induration, and the hand becomes completely fixed in a partially flexed position.

TABLE 3.1

Reflex Sympathetic Dystrophy	
Major	**Minor**
Causalgia	Post-fracture
	Post-cerebrovascular accident
Phantom pain	Post-myocardial infarction
Thalamic syndrome	Post-injection
	Post-casting
	Post-sprain

Treatment

Treatment of the shoulder-hand-finger syndrome involves:

- Initial recognition;
- Emerging the entire hand in ice for brief periods (1 to 2 minutes as tolerated);
- Active and passive elevation of the total arm above the heart level for most of the day;
- Active and passive exercises of the glenohumeral joint to increase the range of motion;
- Active and passive range-of-motion exercises of all the joints of the wrist and fingers; and
- Vasoconstrictive dressing of the fingers distal to proximal wrapping of the fingers with strings, which then are released and reapplied until the edema is gone.

REFLEX SYMPATHETIC DYSTROPHY

A painful shoulder that impairs function without specific involvement of the hand may also initiate the shoulder-hand-finger syndrome. There are numerous conditions descriptive of CRPS that include the shoulder-hand-finger syndrome with resultant similar painful syndromes. Bonica[5] divided these syndromes into major and minor (Table 3.1). Shoulder-hand-finger syndrome falls into the category of minor.

Unlike in reflex sympathetic dystrophy (RSD) and CRPS, the sympathetic nervous system may be initially absent in shoulder-hand-finger syndrome, although it may be the primary causative factor. This was noted by Moberg,[6] who based his opinion on the fact that this syndrome is rarely seen in people younger than 40 years old, which is when sympathetic nervous system involvement is the most prominent.[7]

REFERENCES

1. MacConnaill MA. Studies in the mechanics of synovial joints. *Irish J Med Sci.* 1946;21:223.

2. Harden RN, Baron R, Janig W, eds. *Complex Regional Pain Syndrome: Progress in Pain Research and Management.* Seattle, Wash: International Association for the Study of Pain; 2001.

3. Davies PM. *Steps to Follow: A Guide to the Treatment of Adult Hemiplegia.* New York, NY: Springer-Verlag; 1985.

4. Cailliet R. *Shoulder in Hemiplegia.* Philadelphia, Pa: FA Davis; 1980.

5. Bonica JJ. Causalgia and other reflex sympathetic dystrophies. In: *The Management of Pain.* Philadelphia, Pa: Lea & Febiger; 1953.

6. Moberg E. The shoulder-hand-finger syndrome as a whole. *Surg Clin North Am.* 1960;40:367.

7. Davis SW, Petrillo CR, Eichberg RD, Chu DS. Shoulder-hand-finger syndrome in a hemiplegic population: a five-year retrospective study. *Arch Phys Med Rehabil.* 1977;58:353–356.

chapter 4

Elbow Complex

The elbow complex is made up of the joints between the distal humerus and the proximal ulna and radius bones. The ulna articulates within the trochlear groove of the humerus, and the radial head articulates on the convex capitulum (Figure 4.1).

Elbow flexion and extension occur between the ulna and the humerus, and pronation-supination (rotation) occurs between the head of the radius and the capitulum of the humerus.

The trochlea of the proximal ulna and the capitulum of the lateral condyle of the humerus are coated with articular cartilage, as is the

FIGURE 4.1

Elbow Complex A, Posterior view of extended elbow. Ulnar (U; olecranon process) is inserted into fossa of humerus (H). Radius (R) rotates (pronates [P]) and supinates (S) about capitulum (CAP) of medial aspect of humerus. ME indicates medial epicondyle; LE, lateral epicondyle. B, Anterior view of elbow complex in which ulna (U) is divided by a ridge fitting into fossa. H indicates humerus; R, radius; P, pronation; and S, supination. C, Side view showing insertion of ulna (U) into fossa of humerus (H) on extension (E). F indicates flexion; R, radius.

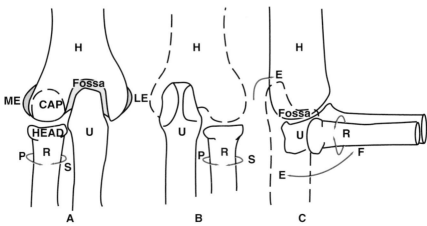

FIGURE 4.2

Ligaments of Elbow Complex A, Medial ligaments attach from medial epicondyles (ME) to ulna (U) and radius (R). Radial-ulnar articulation rotates about annular ligament (AL). H indicates humerus. B, Ligaments originating from lateral epicondyle (LE) attach to ulna. H indicates humerus.

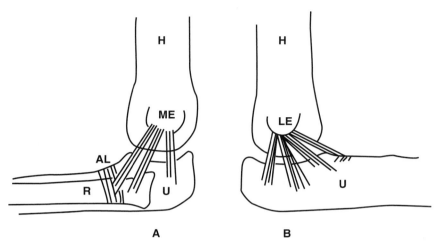

head of the radius. The head of the radius rotates on the inner aspect of the ulna by the annular ligament. The humeroulnar, humeroradial, and radioulnar joints are enclosed within a single capsule. The stability of the elbow complex is furnished by the medial and lateral collateral ligaments (Figure 4.2).

The medial collateral ligament is triangular and connects the medial epicondyle to the ulna, and the lateral ligament, also fan shaped, extends from the lateral epicondyle and attaches to the annular ligament, which encircles the head of the radius.

AXIS OF MOTION OF ELBOW COMPLEX

Flexion and extension occur through the middle of the trochlea around a longitudinal axis through the shaft of the humerus. When flexed to 90 degrees, the angle is termed the carrying angle. The forearm rotates about the capitulum through approximately 145 degrees.

Flexion is activated by the brachial muscle, which inserts close to the axis of rotation. The brachial muscle is greatest dependent on the angulation of flexion and is not influenced by the degree of pronation or supination of the forearm. The musculus biceps brachii also attaches close to the axis of rotation and is greatest at approximately 90 degrees of elbow flexion. It is a supinator by its attachment to the radius. Extension of the forearm is by the triceps.

PATHOMECHANICS

Injury to the elbow complex is usually external trauma that exceeds the normal range of motion of the ulnohumeral or the radial-ulnar joints. Any force that exceeds the resistance of the collateral ligaments also causes impairment.

EPICONDYLITIS

The most common elbow pain and impairment occur from the muscles that attach to the epicondyles of the humerus. The attachments of these muscles are to the periosteum of the condyles and, when injured, cause a condition termed *epicondylitis*.[1-3]

TENNIS ELBOW: LATERAL EPICONDYLITIS

History

Due to the prevalence of athletic activities, there is an inflammation at the site of origin of the extensor muscles at the lateral epicondyle from repeated forceful contraction of the wrist extensor muscles, primarily the extensor carpi radialis brevis. Medial epicondylitis (not usually called "tennis elbow") is caused by forceful repetitive contraction of the musculi pronator teres, flexor carpi radialis, and flexor carpi ulnaris. These injuries are considered tendinitis, but there is also usually some displacement of the periosteum from the bone where the tendons attach.

Clinically, there is exquisite tenderness over the affected epicondyle and the aggravation of the pain from active contraction of the involved muscles. In lateral epicondylitis, or "tennis elbow," the tenderness is over the lateral epicondyle and is aggravated by extension of the wrist and fingers.

The impairment is considered to be a tearing of the muscle attachments to the periosteum of the condyle. Small tears may occur within the body of the muscles near their tendinous attachments, which are opened on contraction of the finger muscles with simultaneous wrist extension.

Confirmation and relief of pain may be verified by injecting procaine hydrochloride or a derivative and a soluble steroid into the area. Manipulation of the tennis elbow completes the tear, and then emergence from a deformed or narrowed foramen in the cervical spine partially denervates the nerve. When the nerve is inflamed, it sends myopathic impulses to the muscles innervated by the specific myotomes—in this case the muscles attaching to one of the epicondyles to reunite in a stable condition.

Diagnosis

Patients who present with symptoms and findings of lateral epicondylitis usually complain of pain in the elbow on the lateral side upon gripping or wrist extension while gripping an object. They also complain of weakness in the elbow due to the pain.

Clinically there is localized tenderness. The pain is aggravated or caused by manually resisting wrist extension and gripping. Passive flexion of the forearm with the hand flexed often reproduces the symptoms as does forceful flexion of the wrist with simultaneous extension and pronation of the forearm.

Radiological tests are not revealing as the pathology is all in the soft tissues where the extensor muscles attach to the periosteum of the epicondyle.

Treatment

Immobilizing the elbow or splinting it to prevent extension and flexion is effective. The splint must encircle the forearm and must extend to prevent any wrist motion. The fingers from the metacarpals are left free to permit manipulation.

Local injection of lidocaine hydrochloride and steroid into the area of tenderness is beneficial. Dry needling of the area has its proponents. Ergonomic exercises have also been proposed.[4,5] Manipulation to forcefully tear the attachment of the extensor muscle group from the periosteum has also been proposed. Surgical intervention should be considered as a last resort.

FIGURE 4.3

Cubital Tunnel Ulnar nerve is contained within olecranon fossa of humerus. Sensory and motor branches of ulnar nerve within cubital canal are shown. Pronated forearm exposes direct pressure on nerve.

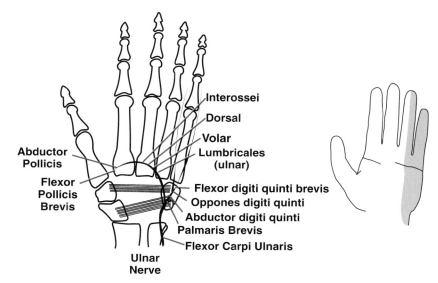

NEUROPATHOLOGY OF ELBOW COMPLEX

History

Of all the peripheral nerves of the brachial plexus at the elbow complex, the ulnar nerve is the most prominent and the most vulnerable to direct trauma. The ulnar nerve is contained within the olecranon groove made into the cubital tunnel by the arcuate ligament (Figure 4.3).

Superficial prominence of this nerve occurs when the forearm is pronated. Because the sensory portion of the ulnar nerve is more superficial, sensory symptoms are noted earlier from pressure of trauma. Symptoms of ulnar nerve compression are paresthesia (numbness or tingling) in the dermatomic distribution of the ulnar nerve in the hand. This is the ulnar half of the fourth finger and the entire fifth finger.

Diagnosis

The differential diagnosis is to determine whether the symptoms occur as a result of ulnar nerve pressure at the elbow or from neuropathy due to cervical discogenic disease, thoracic outlet compression, or ulnar nerve pressure at the wrist. Diagnosis also involves testing all of the muscles supplied by the ulnar nerve and objectively confirming the diagnosis electromyographically.

Treatment

Conservative management is to avoid direct pressure on the nerve during activities of daily living, as recovery is usually noted if pressure is avoided. This avoidance is best accomplished by the patient wearing a sponge pad over the cubital tunnel and avoiding excessive elbow flexion and pronation. Surgical decompression may be needed, but nerve transplantation away from the olecranon fossa often fails, because it exposes the nerve to direct pressure from its changed position and protection within the fossa.[6,7]

RADIAL NERVE COMPRESSION

History

The radial nerve, in its passage through the elbow complex, may become entrapped. As the nerve passes the lateral epicondyle of the humerus, it divides into a superficial branch and a deep branch, which is the origin of the musculus extensor carpi radialis.

Forceful repeated contraction of the extensor carpi radialis (wrist extension in the radial direction), extensor digitorum communis (extension of the fingers), and the extensor carpi ulnaris (extension of the wrist in an ulnar direction), can cause compression of the radial nerve, as these actions cause tightening of the fibrous band.

Diagnosis

The symptoms of radial nerve compression are paresthesia (numbness and tingling) in the dermatomic area of the radial nerve. It can often be initiated or aggravated by manual pressure of the forearm muscles over the nerve. If compression persists, weakness of the muscles innervated by the radial nerve occurs. This weakness is detected by testing supination of the forearm, finger extension, wrist extension, and abduction of the thumb. Electromyographic and nerve conduction studies confirm the diagnosis.

Treatment

Release of the compression may require surgical intervention and should be followed by a period of splinting the arm and wrist in a neutral position. However, splinting should not be prolonged to prevent permanent paresis from the compression.

SKELETAL TRAUMA TO ELBOW

History

Any hyperextension of the elbow complex can impinge the head of the ulna within the olecranon fossa, with subluxation of the ulna and damage to the entrapped capsule and the cartilage of the joint. There is limited and painful extension of the elbow.

Trauma also may cause dislocation of the radial head within the annular fibers as well as local tenderness and painful supination-pronation of the forearm. Skeletal trauma to the elbow is diagnosed by radiologic studies.[8]

Diagnosis

The history of the injury to the elbow is important to verify the hyperextension that occurred. Demonstrating the maneuver to the patient may improve the patient's memory of the injury and while doing this maneuver gently, the pain may be reproduced. The range of motion must be compared to the opposite arm. Palpation of the radial head may reveal a separation or a fracture, in which case radiological studies will reveal the site and extent of the injury.

Treatment

Treatment is determined by the type and extent of the injury. In a fracture, passive or open reduction is necessary to realign the fragments.

REFERENCES

1. Gunn CC, Milbrandt WE. Tennis elbow and the cervical spine. *Can Med Assoc J*. 1976;l114(9):803–809.

2. Gunn CC, Milbrandt WE, Little AS, Mason KE. Dry needling of muscle motor points for chronic low back pain: a randomized clinical trial with long-term follow-up. *Spine*. 1980;5:279–291.

3. Nirschi RP. Muscle and tendon trauma: tennis elbow. In: Morrey BF, ed. *The Elbow and its Disorders*. Philadelphia, Pa: WB Saunders Co; 1985.

4. Bowling RW, Rockar P. The elbow complex. In: Goulde JA, Davies GJ, eds. *Orthopedic and Sorts Physical Therapy*. St. Louis, Mo: Mosby; 1985.

5. Kivi P. The etiology and conservative treatment of humeral epicondylitis. *Scand J Rehab Med*. 1983;15:37–41.

6. Reddy MP. Ulnar nerve entrapment syndrome at the elbow. *Orthop Rev*. 1983;12:69.

7. Payan J. Anterior transportation of the ulnar nerve: an electrophysiological study. *J Neurol Neurosurg Psychiatry*. 1970;33:157–165.

8. Conway RR, Tanner ED. Elbow pain. In: Kaplan PE, Tanner ED, eds. *Musculoskeletal Pain and Disability*. Norwalk, Conn: Appleton & Lange; 1989.

Wrist Complex

The wrist performs the most complex motion of any joint in the body in placing the hand where daily functions are needed. The loss of any one of its conjoined functions—extension-flexion, circumduction, or rotation—greatly impairs hand-finger activities.

Clinically, the wrist is subject to fracture, strains, and sprains from falls on the extended hand. Besides causing impairment and pain of the wrist and subsequent limitation of movement, trauma can also damage vital organs at the wrist. These organs include the median nerve, ulnar nerve, radial and ulnar arteries, and tendons of the forearm that move the fingers (Figure 5.1).

The wrist complex gains stability from the joint capsules but primarily depends on the wrist ligaments for support. These ligaments are subject to strain, elongation, and degrees of disruption in sprain injuries. *Sprain* implies that a joint has been moved beyond its physiological limits, causing damage to the capsule, ligaments, and even tendons of that joint.[1]

The radiocarpal joint moves predominately by sliding of the carpals on the radius and the radioulnar disk. Because of the convex surface of the carpus on the concave surfaces of the radial and ulnar bones, the slide occurs in a direction opposite to the movement of the hand. The ligaments normally check each slide at the end of their range and become strained or sprained when exceeded.

Ligaments, which are used to connect one bony component to another, are composed of dense fibrous tissue, of which collagen is major component. These ligaments have the tensile strength of steel. Collagen fibers are nonelastic, but their arrangement allows some deformation.[2]

Wrist Bones and Organs in their Proximity Bones forming the wrist joint are radius (R), ulna (U), scaphoid (S), lunate (L), and triquetral (T). Pisiform (P), hamate (H), and capitate (C) bones are second row of hand bones. Vessels and nerves in proximity of wrist bones also are shown.

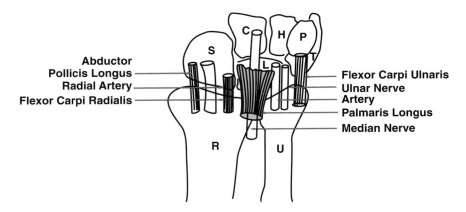

SPRAIN

A sprain is excessive elongation of the capsules and ligaments around the joint without disruption or avulsion of any of the involved tissues.

History

A patient recalls an injury, a fall or an external force that moved the wrist past its normal range of motion. This causes excessive elongation of the capsules and ligaments around the joint without disruption or avulsion of any of the involved tissues.

Diagnosis

Immediately after the injury there occurs swelling, discoloration, deformation of the wrist, tenderness, and painful active and passive motion of the joint. Normal activities of the hand are not possible. Radiological studies are normal.

Treatment

Initial treatment involves the application of ice to prevent further swelling and possible bleeding. Further treatment involves splinting for comfort while normal healing occurs. Local application of ice decreases swelling, tenderness, and the pain of movement but must be followed by heat to ensure healing and restoration of normal function.

As soon as tolerated, passive and then active range-of-motion exercises restore normal function and the strength of the involved muscles. Normal function is expected unless the force has been so excessive as to tear the ligaments, capsule, tendons, or dislocated the bones, which would be apparent through x-ray studies. In such cases, direct treatment at correcting these defects.

DISLOCATIONS

History

A dislocation is the temporary displacement of a bone from its normal position in a joint, which exceeds a sprain.[3] Most dislocations occur as an impact of a fall on the extended arm and the wrist in hyperextension. The most common carpal dislocation is of the lunate moving around the rest of the carpus.

Diagnosis

In dislocation of the wrist, the wrist appears deformed dependent upon the direction and the extent of the dislocation as revealed by radiological studies. Active gentle mobilization of the wrist reveals the excessive range of motion now possible as compared to the other wrist.

Treatment

Upon radiologic diagnosis, the dislocation is manually reduced through a process called "closed reduction." The wrist is placed in a plaster cast in the neutral position for 8 weeks. Upon removal of the cast, the wrist is treated with assisted exercises to regain normal range of motion and strengthen the ligaments and capsule. If closed reduction is not possible, an open reduction with pinning may be needed.

COLLES FRACTURE

History

Colles fracture is the most common osseous injury of the wrist joint and follows from a fall on the outstretched hand with either dorsal or radial displacement of the distal fragment. It resembles what has been termed the "silver fork" deformity.

Diagnosis

The clinical diagnosis is a painful deformed distal radius after a fall upon the extended arm. The site and extent of the deformity must be confirmed radiologically as to type and severity. The distal radius fragment has usually moved dorsally and outward, causing impaired wrist motion and often impaired function of the tendons that pass the fracture site.

Diagnostically the impaired wrist function must also include a careful examination of possible impaired circulation and nerve function that has resulted from the fracture.

Treatment

Treatment of a Colles fracture is dictated by the severity of the fracture and any complicating factors, which may include the median nerve. If the median nerve is compressed, it must be decompressed immediately.

Minimally displaced and noncomminuted fractures (termed Type I or II) can be treated by closed reduction followed by plaster casting with the wrist placed in 10- to 20-degree flexion and 15-degree ulnar deviation. It is mandatory that the casting permit movement of the fingers at the metacarpal-phalangeal joints distally and that these joints be actively moved repeatedly during healing of the fracture. The shoulder and elbow also must be actively and passively moved through complete range of motion.

Unstable fractures or radial fractures that fail to heal must have surgical intervention.

CARPAL TUNNEL SYNDROME

History

"What is carpal tunnel syndrome?" An editorial in *JAMA* posed this question.[4] It was stated in that article that carpal tunnel syndrome (CTS) is a common diagnosis with a lifetime risk of 10% and an annual incidence of 0.1% among adults.[5,6] The prevalence of CTS in the general population is 6.0% in men and 5.8% in women. More than 200,000 surgical procedures for CTS release are performed every year in the United States.

Brain and colleagues[7] were the first to report the pathological basis for the syndrome, which is an increased pressure within the carpal tunnel (Figure 5.2) and interference with perfusion of the median nerve (Figure 5.3), with resultant numbness, tingling, and gradual weakness.

FIGURE 5.2

Ligaments of Carpal Tunnel A, Distal ligament extends from tubercle (TUB) of trapezium (Tp) to hook of hamate (H). Proximal ligament from tubercle of scaphoid (S) to pisiform bone (P). L indicates lunate and MC, metacarpal bone. B, Carpal bones of carpal tunnel (CT) are scaphoid (S), capitate (CT), hamate (H), triquetral (Tq), and pisiform (P). Within ligaments are flexor carpi radialis tendon (FCR), flexor carpi ulnaris (FCU), blood vessels (BV), and ulnar nerve (UN). Medial nerve (MN) is within canal. C, Piriformis (P) is a sesmoid bone within tendon of flexor carpi ulnaris (FCU), which attaches to base of fifth metacarpal bone (MC) and hook of hamate (HH). When muscles tense, transverse ligament (TL) also tenses.

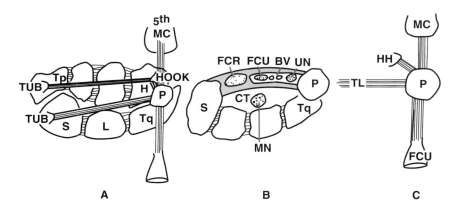

FIGURE 5.3

Median Nerve Dermatomic area supplied by median nerve (MN) is shown. Muscles innervated by median nerve are flexor pollicis brevis (FPB), opponens pollicis (OP), and abductor pollicis brevis (APB). 1L and 2L indicate first and second lumbricals; DTL, distal transverse ligament; and PTL, proximal transverse ligament. These nerves are not shown: flexor pollicis longus, flexor digitorum sublimis, flexor digitorum profundus, flexor carpi radialis, pronator quadratus, pronator teres, and palmaris longus, as they are all supplied by the median nerve.

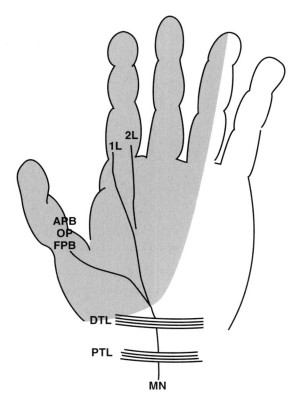

Diagnosis

Median nerve compression has been considered a repetitive strain injury in occupations that require the wrist being repeatedly flexed and extended with simultaneous finger flexion. In magnetic resonance imaging (MRI) studies during wrist extension, the median nerve becomes flattened in the sagittal plane and movement is decreased as it lies close to the flexor retinaculum.[8] In wrist flexion, the nerve moves transversely in a radial direction. Increased intratunnel pressure causes a substantial decrease in these motions. Standard electrophysiological studies to confirm median nerve compression at the wrist are 0.8 milliseconds median-to-ulnar peak latency in conduction velocity testing.

Clinically the patient complains of numbness and tingling of the fingers (usually the index and inner second fingers) innervated by the median nerve. Weakness is also common in the muscles innervated—weakness in opposing and abducting the thumb, and ultimately atrophy of the thenar eminence.

Treatment

Conservative treatment involves the avoidance of making fist or finger flexion with sustained wrist extension and taking frequent work breaks.

Exercises are recommended. One exercise routine includes the following (H. Seradge, MD, unpublished data, 1996):

1. Stand with arms relaxed at the side.
2. Raise an arm to shoulder level with forearm supinated and hand facing up. Spread fingers and extend finger toward the floor.
3. Make a fist and flex hand at the wrist.
4. Flex elbow and bring hand toward shoulder.
5. With the arm-hand in that position, externally rotate the arm and turn the head toward the flexed hand.
6. Straighten elbow and fingers and extend the wrist toward the floor, then rotate the head away from the extended arm.
7. Bring both arms to shoulder level and place both flexed wrists against each other with fingers extended.
8. At shoulder level extend both hand and fingers; bring them together and slowly elevate the hand over the head.
9. Bring both hands behind the head.
10. Abduct both arms at shoulder level with wrists flexed in a fist.
11. With fingers straightened and wrists extended, bring both arms behind the waist.

Ergonomic advice is indicated, as it is apparent that repetitive motion requiring wrist extension and simultaneous repeated finger flexion is a causative factor in this condition. Although all causative factors have not been confirmed, it stands to reason that frequent periods of rest from daily occupational activities should be encouraged, along with exercises such as those just mentioned.

A recent article by Wilgis[9] in evaluating the treatment outcomes for carpal tunnel syndrome concluded that surgical decompression is advisable rather than a prolonged period of conservative treatment, which offers limited benefit. Gerritsen et al[10] stated that after a review of outcomes after 18 months of treatment with a splint, surgical decompression was more desirable. In the short term, splinting was favored, but after 18 months, splinting was effective in only 37% of patients, whereas surgery was effective in 94%. Recurrence was prominent in the conservatively treated patients, whereas recurrence was essentially not found in those surgically treated. These findings suggest that the treatment protocol should include a temporal factor; after a period of conservative treatment deemed unsuccessful on the basis of objective findings, surgical intervention should be considered in less than 12 months.

ULNAR NERVE COMPRESSION

History

The ulnar nerve is subjected to compression at the wrist as well as at the elbow. At the wrist, it enters the hand in a shallow trough between the pisiform bone and the hook of the hamate in what is called Guyon canal. The roof of this tunnel is the volar carpal ligament and the musculus palmaris longus. Only 2 terminal branches of the ulnar nerve run in the canal.

The superficial branch of the palmar branch innervates the musculus palmaris brevis and the palmar and dorsal skin of the fifth finger and the ulnar half of the fourth finger. The deep branch innervates the following: the hypothenar muscles, 2 lateral lumbrical muscles, all the interosseous muscles, and the musculi adductor pollicis and flexor pollicis brevis.

Diagnosis

Diagnosis consists of a history of difficulty in hand grasping, paresthesia of the ulnar sensory nerve distribution, loss of pinch strength of the thumb, and gradual atrophy of the interosseous muscles. There can be a Tinel sign to tapping the ulnar nerve at the wrist. Diagnostic electromyography (EMG) should be used for confirmation.

Treatment

Treatment involves avoiding all activities that have been discovered as causing the condition. Splinting and steroid injections into the tunnel are usually effective. The exercises advised for the median nerve have not been specifically advocated for ulnar neuropathy, but they may be valuable. If conservative treatment is ineffectual, surgical intervention is indicated.

REFERENCES

1. Norkin CC, Levangie PK. *Joint Structure and Function*. Philadelphia, Pa: FA Davis Co; 1983.
2. Widmann FK. *Pathobiology: How Disease Happens*. Boston, Mass: Little, Brown & Co; 1978.
3. Stanley BG, Tribuzi SM, eds. *Concepts in Hand Rehabilitation*. Philadelphia, Pa: FA Davis Co; 1992.
4. Franzblau A, Werner RA. What is carpal tunnel syndrome? *JAMA*. 1999; 282:186-187.
5. Stevens JC, Sun S, Beard CM, O'Fallon WM, Kurland LT. Carpal tunnel syndrome in Rochester, Minnesota, 1961 to 1980. *Neurology*. 1988;38: 134-138.
6. Quality Standards Subcommittee of the American Academy of Neurology. Practice parameters for carpal tunnel syndrome. *Neurology*. 1993;43: 2406-2409.
7. Brain WR, Wright AD, Wilkinson M. Spontaneous compression of both median nerves at the carpal tunnel: six cases treated surgically. *Lancet*. 1947;1:277-282.
8. Greening J, Smart S, Leary R, Hall-Craggs M, O'Higgins P, Lynn B. Reduced movement of median nerve in carpal tunnel during wrist flexion in patients with non-specific arm pain. *Lancet*. 1999;354:217-218.
9. Wilgis EF. Treatment options for carpal tunnel syndrome. *JAMA*. 2002; 288:1281-1282.
10. Gerritsen AA, de Vet HC, Scholten RJ, Betelsmann FW, de Krom MC, Bouter LM. Splinting vs surgery in the treatment of carpal tunnel syndrome: a randomized controlled trial. *JAMA*. 2002;288:1245-1251.

chapter 6

Fingers

Tendonitis is a common source of pain and impaired function of the fingers of the hand.[1] The histopathoanatomical factors leading to tendinitis remain obscure, but many of the factors include fibrocytic proliferation, thickening, collagen fiber breakdown, and even adherence to contiguous tissues.[2-4]

The extensor tendons of the fingers are susceptible to injury, because they are superficial with little overlying protective tissues other than skin. Flexor tendon injuries are more tenuous, as they are located in what is termed "no man's land" (Figure 6.1).

MALLET FINGER

History

The distal phalanx is extended by the superficial extensor tendon. A flexion force against the extended finger can rupture this tendon. Most tears occur where the tendon inserts on the phalanx, but some 25% have an avulsion of the bone to which the tendon inserts.

Diagnosis

After injury to the hand, a tear in the extensor tendon may occur at the middle phalanx, causing the distal phalanx to droop. Clinically, the distal phalanx remains flexed and cannot be actively extended. The resulting deformity is termed a "boutonniere" deformity.

Treatment

Conservative treatment consists of a splint that keeps the distal phalanx hyperextended for a period of 5 weeks.

FIGURE 6.1

"No Man's Land" Profundus tendon attaches to distal phalanx and is enclosed within division of superficialis tendon that attaches to middle phalanx. Both profundus and sublimis flexor tendons are tightly enclosed within a sheath, and surgical repair is fraught with failure.[5]

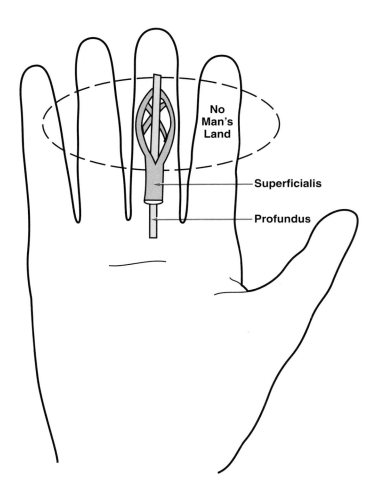

RUPTURE OF EXTENSOR POLLICIS LONGUS TENDON

History

The extensor pollicis longus tendon curves around the dorsal radial tubercle of Lister and continues to insert on the thumb. It is the lateral tendon of the "snuffbox," palpable at the distal wrist made prominent by extending the thumb against resistance.

Diagnosis

Clinically, the patient cannot extend the distal joint of the thumb and has weakness in extending the proximal joint of the thumb. The normal tendon usually can be palpated when the thumb is actively extended.

Treatment

Primary suturing of the torn tendon is not feasible as the suturing will not hold nor is the repaired tendon functional. A graft may be necessary following which holding the corrected thumb is necessary for 1 month.[6] This splint is a plaster or plastic splint placed on the dorsum and palmar surface of the thumb, holding all joints in slight extension.

DE QUERVAIN DISEASE

History

Tenosynovitis of the thumb abductor longus and the pollicis brevis at the radiostyloid process, where they are enclosed under a synovially lined ligament, commonly causes an adhesive tendinitis. The condition is known as de Quervain disease.

Diagnosis

Signs and symptoms include swelling and pain over the radial styloid process, which is aggravated by forceful ulnar deviation of the wrist with the thumb flexed and abducted. This maneuver is known as the Finkelstein test.[5]

Numerous tendinitis conditions occur, such as extensor pollicis longus tendinitis, extensor indicis proprius tendinitis, extensor digiti minimi tendinitis, and extensor carpi ulnaris tendinitis. All of these conditions exhibit tenderness over the specific tendon and are aggravated by extension of that tendon.

Treatment

Splinting has been advocated to prevent further contracture but is very difficult. Local injection of a steroid into the distal end of the compartment is also beneficial. Surgical release of the contracture has been suggested, but to date has been met with disappointing results.

TRIGGER FINGERS

History

Snapping of the flexor tendons that is felt and heard during active finger flexion and/or reextension is termed "trigger fingers." These snapping tendons allegedly occur from repeated trauma to the flexor tendon, which results in thickening of the flexor sheath and formation of a nodule. When this nodule passes the tranverse annular ligament, it snaps. If the nodule increases in size or the annular ligament thickens, the nodule cannot pass the annular fiber and the finger remains locked in the flexed position (Figure 6.2).

Diagnosis

A trigger finger is suspected when flexing a finger causes a snapping that may be heard or felt. Full flexion may initially be denied and the finger remains flexed only to gradually reextend. In more severe and recurrent triggers, the finger remains flexed and may defy active and passive extension.

Treatment

Conservative treatment consists of injecting an analgesic agent and steroid into the sheath. Usually a single injection will succeed, but a second injection is indicated if symptoms persist. Failure to succeed requires surgical resection of the transverse ligament.

FIGURE 6.2

Trigger Fingers Site of nodule in flexor tendon that becomes a "trigger" or snaps when it passes under the annular ligament during finger flexion.

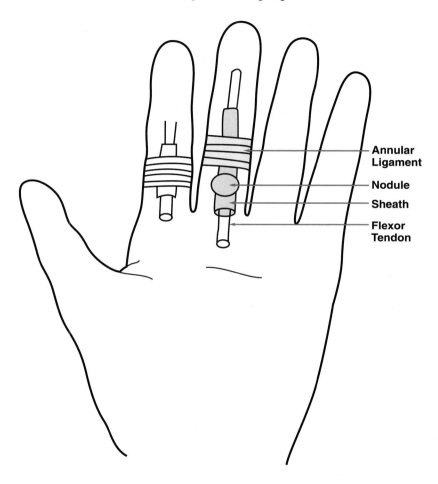

Annular
Ligament

Nodule

Sheath

Flexor
Tendon

DUPUYTREN CONTRACTURE

History

Dupuytren contracture is a fibrous contracture of the palmar fascia with gradual flexion contracture of the finger flexors at the metacarpal-phalangeal or proximal interphalangeal joints. The causative factors remain unknown, but originally it was found in white men in their fifth to seventh decades of life. The condition rarely occurs in women. Vocational repetitive trauma is no longer considered a factor.

The fascia of the hand is a continuance of the palmaris longus tendon, which normally proceeds distally to attach to the sides of the proximal and middle phalanges. The overlying skin is thin, has scant subcutaneous fat, and is connected to the fascia by small fasciculi. The deep fascial sheath proceeds deeper to form septa forming 8 longitudinal compartments that contain the flexor tendons, the lumbrical muscles, and the associated neurovascular bundles.

The palmar fascia receives its blood supply from tiny branches of the superficial arch of the distal radial and ulnar arteries that penetrate the fascia. As the fascia thickens, it contracts, pulling on the overlying skin and causing "dimples." Gradually, as the fascia thickens, it occludes the blood vessels, causing more fibrous tissue and more flexor contraction of the fingers.

Diagnosis

Clinically, Dupuytren contracture is a painless thickening of the palmar skin and underlying tissues with some dimpling. The initial site is close to the distal palmar crease near the ring fingers, with bilateral involvement in 40% of cases. Flexion contracture usually occurs at the metacarpal-phalangeal joints. Four stages have been defined:

1. A nodule of the palmar fascia that does not include the overlying skin.
2. A nodule in the fascia that includes the overlying skin.
3. Findings as in stage 2 but with some flexion contracture of 1 or more fingers.
4. Findings as in stage 3 but with both tendon and joint contracture.

The stage is not of therapeutic significance until there is impairment of vital finger function that impairs activities of daily living.

Treatment

Treatment remains limited in value and consists of injection of trypsin, chymotrypsin, hyaluronidase, and lidocaine into the contracture, followed by passive stretching of the involved fingers. Substantial improvement or at least maintenance of the degree of contraction delays the need for surgery, which has limited value.

SPRAINS AND DISLOCATIONS

History

Sprain implies an excessive force that causes subluxation of a joint and soft-tissue damage to the capsule, ligaments, and tendons. Radiographs may be unrevealing when the subluxation has been reduced, but a thorough physical examination may reveal that soft-tissue injuries have occurred.

Diagnosis

Clinically, there is swelling, local tenderness, pain, and change in joint range of motion compared with the contralateral joint. In a severe subluxation of the metacarpal-phalangeal joint, the palmar plate may be torn. These plates are fibrocatilagenous plates that reinforce the capsule by limiting hyperextension. The plate has 2 component tissues. The proximal portion is cartilaginous and the distal is membranous. The distal portion is firmly attached to the phalanx, whereas the proximal cartilaginous portion is loosely attached and can be severed by a forceful extension of the joint. Prolonged immobilization of the joint in flexion allows the membranous portion to retract, leading to a flexion contracture of the finger.

Treatment

In a mild sprain/strain, when there has been no disruption of the capsule, ligaments, or tendons, temporarily splinting the part will be effective. At first, local ice application to prevent inflammation or microscopic hemorrhage is indicated. Later, local heat to the part with exercises to regain flexibility and strength restores function.

If there has been a dislocation, the parts dislocated must be restored manually to their normal alignment. Then, depending on the severity, the joint must be splinted until healing. If severe dislocation has occurred, surgical intervention may be needed.

THUMB

History

The carpometacarpal joint of the thumb is an articulation between the first metacarpal and the trapezium. It is a saddle joint permitting flexion-extension, abduction-adduction, and some degree of axial rotation. The capsule of the thumb carpometacarpal joint is relatively lax, allowing a greater range of motion than is permitted in other joints. Opposition is vital for prehension and is a combination of abduction, adduction, and flexion of the first metacarpal joint with some degree of rotation. The joint is essentially 2 saddle joints.

Diagnosis

Dislocation of the thumb with or without tearing of the capsule is one of the most common dislocations of the hand. The most frequent injury to the thumb is due to hyperextension. It is diagnosed clinically by visual and manual methods and is verified radiologically. Treatment is by traction reduction and immobilization in a plaster cast for 3 to 4 weeks.

Recurrent dislocations may be followed by contracture, which may require capsulotomy. The thumb joint, by being exposed to frequent injuries and repetitive stresses, may be a site of degenerative arthritis. This is suspected by pain and crepitation and is verified radiologically. Treatment, when severe and disabling, is by fusions, orthosis replacement, or both.

Treatment

A dislocated thumb presents a significant approach as the joint is multidirectional and includes rotation as well as flexion, extension, and abduction. Appropriate splinting in a mild sprain is often effective, but after dislocation surgical opinion is required, as the thumb is vital in all hand/finger activities. Reduction and splinting awaiting consultation is indicated.

REFERENCES

1. Cailliet R. *Hand Pain and Impairment*. 4th ed. Philadelphia, Pa: FA Davis Co; 1994.

2. Rigby BJ, Horai N, Spikes JD. The mechanical behavior of rattail tendon. *J Gen Physiol*. 1959;43:265-283.

3. Warren CG, Lehmann JF, Koblanski JN. Elongation of rat tail tendon: effect of load and temperature. *Arch Phys Med Rehabil*. 1971;52:465-474.

4. Tillman LJ, Cummings CG. Biological mechanisms of connective tissue mutability: In: Currier DP, Nelson RM, eds. *Dynamics of Human Biological Tissues*. Philadelphia, Pa: FA Davis Co; 1992.

5. Finkelstein HJ. Stenosing tenosynovaginitis at the radial styloid process. *J Bone Joint Surg*. 1930;12:509.

6. Byrne JJ. *The Hand: Its Anatomy and Diseases*. Springfield, Ill: Charles C Thomas Publishers; 1959.

chapter 7

Foot-Ankle Impairment

Any injury or disease that compromises function of the foot and ankle impairs locomotion. Because the ankle is a ligament, supported joint injury to any ligament will contribute to instability and impairment. Ankle stability is decreased when the foot is plantar flexed, because in that position the narrow portion of the talus is between the malleoli, rendering the joint unstable. Most sports-related ankle sprains are sustained when the athlete is up on the toes and twisted inward. This position stresses the anterior talofibular ligament, which is strained, partially torn, or avulsed from the fibular end (Figure 7.1).

The history of the traumatic event, told by either the patient or an observer, provides the pathomechanism of the injury. As previously stated, the most common injury is to the anterior talofibular ligament, which occurs when the inverted plantar flexed foot is strained. The next most frequent injury is to the calcaneofibular ligament. Because the medial ligaments are more resilient, they are the least injured, with avulsion of the tip of the tibia being the injury sustained.

SPRAINS

Ankle sprains are classified as to severity, completeness, and joint stability, and classification determines the treatment.[1]

First-Degree

Mild, or first-degree, sprains involve a partial tear of the fibers of the ligament without any residual weakness and no instability.

Diagnosis
First-degree sprains exhibit mild swelling and tenderness.

FIGURE 7.1

Ankle Ligaments A, Lateral ligaments of ankle are named by their bony attachments: fibula (F), talus (Ta), and calcaneus (C). Ligaments are anterior talofibular (ATF), posterior talofibular (PTF), calcaneofibular (CF), and talocalcaneal (TC). B. On medial side, there is another bone—navicular (N)—and ligaments are tibial-calcaneal (CT), posterior talotibial (PTT), anterior talotibial (ATT), and tibionavicular (TN).

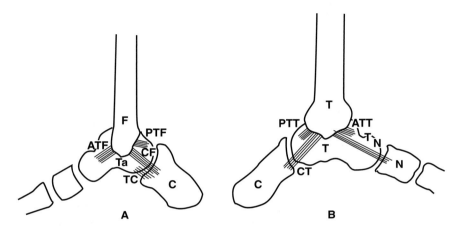

Treatment

This type of sprain responds well to ice application, compression, and elevation. No external support is indicated. Ultimately, strengthening exercises have value.

Second-Degree

Moderate (second-degree) sprains demonstrate an actual tear of a portion of the ligament, but stability of the joint remains.

Diagnosis

Characteristically, there is more severe pain and swelling, ecchymosis, and more tenderness. Some laxity is noted compared with the other ankle.

Treatment

In addition to ice, compression, and elevation, stirrup splints or strapping is indicated. The patient gradually may return to activity with supervision, and exercises are prescribed to regain and maintain the strength and stability of the joint.

The strapping recommended is the Gibney basket-weave adhesive tape method. This taping begins from the medial side of the leg, passes down and under the heel with the foot held in eversion, and then is brought out along the lateral lower aspect of the leg. If there is substantial swelling and tenderness over the lateral malleolus, a cutout foam pad is placed there to minimize local pressure.

Third-Degree

Severe (third-degree) sprains demonstrate a loss of functional stability and imply a complete tear.

Diagnosis

Swelling is extreme, as is ecchymosis. Pain is severe, and manual evidence of instability can be elicited as swelling subsides. In lateral injuries, there is a positive anterior drawer sign (forward sliding of the talus within the mortise).

Treatment

Treatment may require surgical intervention, but healing has been accomplished with conservative nonsurgical care. The decision remains with the physician, the patient, and the need for ultimate stability of the ankle required in an athlete. Post operative care is mandatory and involves strengthening exercises and proprioceptive training with use of a tilt board.[2]

ACHILLES TENDINITIS

History

Inflammation of the Achilles tendon occurs most often from repeated stress of the tendon or from a direct trauma to the tendon. Achilles tendinitis is a frequent sports injury and may occur to the occasional weekend athlete who has a shortened heel cord and has not participated in preventive stretching exercises.

Diagnosis

The findings include a red, warm swelling over the Achilles tendon near its insertion on the calcaneus. Pain can be elicited by having the patient frequently rise up on the toes or having plantar flexion performed against resistance. Crepitation may be elicited from this motion.

Treatment

Therapeutic intervention includes avoidance of the aggravating activities and rest of the injured foot. Local application of ice is indicated. Local steroids can be administered via phonophoresis. A walking cast may be useful if the condition is severe and limiting. After the acute phase subsides, rehabilitation (eg, stretching exercises and strengthening exercises of the gastrocnemius muscle) is valuable.

ACHILLES TENDON TEAR

History

Tearing of the Achilles tendon is rare but severely disabling when it occurs. Tearing occurs most often in sedentary males between ages 30 and 40 who undertake strenuous weekend activities for which they are not physically fit.

Diagnosis

A tear is felt and/or heard, and the person is unable to rise on the toes of that leg. A gap is felt in the tendon in performing the Thompson test, in which the patient is placed prone with both feet over the edge of the examining table and the calves are squeezed. This normally causes the foot to plantar flex but does not occur when the Achilles tendon is severed.

Treatment

Imobilization of the ankle in full plantar flexion often allows the tendon to reattach, heal, and return to function. If surgical repair is considered, it must be undergone early before the collagen fibers of the tendon retract and granulation forms in the gap between fibers. Upon repair, gradual progressive exercises must be initiated to restore full function. Healing is considered to have occurred within 24 months, so a long period of rehabilitation is indicated.

POSTERIOR CALCANEAL BURSITIS

History

There are 2 bursae located in the posterior aspect of the calcaneus that can become inflamed: the retrocalcaneal bursa, which lies between the anterior portion of the Achilles tendon and the adjacent bone, and the calcaneal bursa, which lies between the tendon and the skin. Both or either of these can become inflamed concurrent with Achilles tendinitis due to direct trauma or tight-fitting shoes.

Diagnosis

Pain and tenderness occur over the posterior aspect of the heel and inflammation and swelling may be noted. The bursa can be seen as well as felt. If the bursitis has persisted and become chronic, the skin thickens as well as does the walls of the bursa.

Treatment

Treatment involves initially removing the cause of the bursitis, which often is the offending shoe. Often, cutting out the portion of the heel in the shoe that causes the bursitis is beneficial. A "doughnut" plaster patch over the bursa may decrease the irritation. Aspiration of the bursa may be indicated if it persists and is severe. This may be followed by injecting a steroid or an antibiotic if infection occurs.

CALCANEAL SPURS

History

Plantar (heel) calcaneal spurs and plantar fasciitis occur concurrently and are variations of each other. Both present the same symptoms, have the same mechanism, and are treated in the same manner.

Diagnosis

Plantar fasciitis is inflammation of the plantar fascia where it attaches to the anterior aspect of the calcaneus. It presents as pain noted directly at that site by the patient and is noted on prolonged standing, prolonged walking, and jogging. There is local swelling and tenderness of the anterior undersurface of the calcaneus. Passive dorsiflexion of the toes, where the anterior portion of the fascia attaches, increases the pain by increasing the tension of the fascia. This fascia stabilizes the longitudinal arch and is under more tension in a pronated (flat) foot, which flattens the longitudinal arch.

A spur may develop that at first is asymptomatic and may not be noted in x-ray studies until there is calcification. A spur develops from prolonged excessive traction of the plantar fascia on the

FIGURE 7.2

Formation of Heel Spur Side view of foot shows plantar fascia (PF) attached to calcaneus (C) and stabilizing longitudinal arch. Small figure shows traction on periosteum and ultimate area of spur.

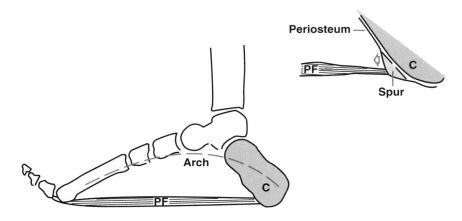

periosteum of the calcaneus with initial inflammation, then bleeding into the avulsed area of the periosteum, with ultimate fibrosis and then calcification (Figure 7.2).

Treatment

Treatment includes attention to the inflammation by initial avoidance of activities that cause pain, local application of ice, oral nonsteroidal anti-inflammatory drugs (NSAIDs), and even injection of an analgesic with a soluble steroid into the area of the spur. This injection enters the area of tenderness and goes to the bone, then is slightly retracted so that the injected fluid enters the space and does not further irritate the bone and its periosteum.

The abnormal condition of the foot that caused the fasciitis must be addressed. If the foot is severely pronated, an orthosis is recommended to supinate the foot and relieve the subtalar pronation. While waiting for the orthosis, taping the ankle and calcaneus in supination is valuable. An inserted heel pad with a cutout over the site of the spurs affords relief.

METATARSALGIA

History

Pain over the heads of the metatarsal bones is a frequent source of foot pain and impairment. Here the patient indicates the exact site of the pain and tenderness by pointing to the undersurfaces of the metatarsal head or heads.

There are several types of metatarsalgia. Primary metatarsalgia is a weight-bearing imbalance of the metatarsal heads due to faulty foot mechanics, such as a severely pronated foot or a short first metatarsal bone causing excessive weight bearing on the second metatarsal head. Secondary metatarsalgia occurs when there is systemic disease such as rheumatoid arthritis or an abnormal gait caused by a stroke or cerebral palsy.

Diagnosis

The diagnosis is made by the presence of tenderness directly over the plantar symptomatic metatarsal head and resulting from manual compression of the head by the examiner. Pressure from the examiner must be directly over the head and not between the heads of adjacent metatarsal bones where the interdigital nerves are located. Pain is noted by the patient at the push-off phase of gait. Often this condition occurs in middle-aged individuals who are in poor physical condition and overweight.

Treatment

Initially, pain relief can be accomplished by soaking the foot in warm water, removal of calluses, and oral NSAID therapy. Treatment is to minimize weight bearing of the afflicted heads. This can be accomplished by the insertion of a pad *behind* the metatarsal heads. "Behind" is stressed because insertion under the heads, to increase the metatarsal arch, increases the pressure on the head.[3] Ultimately, a prosthesis may be needed if a severely pronated foot is considered as an aggravating factor. If the condition is severe and protracted, surgical intervention may be needed.

MORTON NEUROMA

History

Morton neuroma is a painful condition usually occurring between the third and fourth or the second and third metatarsal heads. It is noted after prolonged walking often with ill-fitting shoes that compress the anterior portion of the foot and/or with a high heel. Pain is typically relieved by removing the shoe and massaging the area.

Diagnosis

The examination reveals tenderness between the metatarsal heads. Paresthesia of the 2 adjacent toes may be noted, because the nerve compression is that of the lateral branches of the medial plantar nerve. Manual compression of the forefoot causes the pain, and relief of the pain by injecting an anesthetic agent in the region between the two metatarsal heads confirms the diagnosis.

Treatment

Management requires the patient to remove the compressing footwear, wear a wider shoe, and minimize the height of the heel. Injection of lidocaine and a steroid into the region between the two metatarsal heads inflaming the nerve is effective. If the condition is chronic and resistant to conservative treatment, surgical intervention is indicated, which often reveals a neuroma. Denervating the offending nerve with electrocautery has also been advocated.

HALLUX VALGUS

History

Deformities or inflammation of the big toe are prevalent and disabling. *Hallux valgus*, commonly called a bunion, is probably the most frequent inflammation of the big toe and may be a hereditary condition aggravated by wearing narrow shoes or having degenerative changes of the metatarsal-phalangeal joint (Figure 7.3). Further deformity occurs because of the bowstring effect of the tendon of the extensor hallucis longus and the inability of the musculus abductor hallucis to overcome the deformity aggravated by the adductor hallucis.[4]

FIGURE 7.3
Hallux Valgus (Bunion) First metatarsal bone (1 MT) is in varus compared with normal alignment (dashed line). Proximal phalanx (PP) goes into valgus, causing sesamoids to move laterally. Bunion forms over malaligned metatarsal-phalangeal joint. Degenerative joint changes occur due to this deformity.

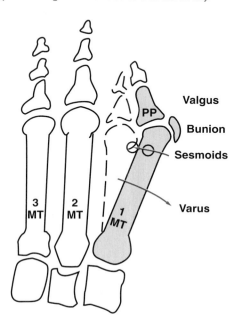

Diagnosis

Pain occurs from the pressure on the medial bony prominence, which inflames the bursa causing it to thicken and ultimately become fibrous. Due to malalignment of the metatarsophalangeal joint, degenerative arthritic changes occur that may lead to hallux rigidus but in the meantime are painful and impairing.

Treatment

Conservative management requires relief of pressure over the bunion site by wearing a corrective shoe with a cutout or by insertion of a felt ring in the shoe. Pain from arthritic changes in the joint may require injection of steroid into the joint as well as oral NSAID therapy and local application of heat or ice.

If pronation is a factor, correction with an orthosis is indicated. Failure to gain relief may suggest surgical intervention. Many surgical techniques have been developed, and a full discussion of them is beyond the scope of this text.[4]

Hallux Rigidus

History

When movement of the metatarsal-proximal phalangeal joint is severely limited or even total, the condition is considered *hallux rigidus*. Any movement of that joint is prevented and alters the normal determinants of gait.[5]

Diagnosis

The patient complains of pain in the area of the big toes and states that the pain occurs at a specific time in the gait, which is heel off when the first toe flexes. When the big toe is examined, the proximal joint has painful crepitation and limited range of motion until the joint becomes totally limited and no motion occurs. Radiological studies reveal the extent of the joint deterioration.

Treatment

Treatment indicates that any motion of the big toe be prevented during gait. This may mean insertion of a steel shank in the shoe that prevents any flexion of the sole.

Before there is complete fusion of the joint, conservative measures should be instituted. These include rest, local application of ice, and injection of steroids in the remaining joint space. A Keller arthroplasty that resects the proximal half of the proximal phalanx may provide relief of pain and improve gait, but it also compromises the propulsion power of gait.[4,5] A rocker-bottom modification to the shoe markedly improves gait and relieves pain.[2]

PES CAVUS

History

An extremely high inflexible longitudinal arch (shown in Figure 7.2) is termed *pes cavus* or *talipes cavus*. There are degrees of flexibility;

in some cases the longitudinal arch depresses on weight bearing to total inflexibility, where there is no change in curvature.[6]

Diagnosis

The increased longitudinal arch places strain on the metatarsal phalangeal joints that must accommodate to the change in gait dynamics causing "clawing" of the toes, uneven distribution of weight bearing over all metatarsal heads, and even shortening of the Achilles tendon. Any of these alone cause pain and impairment and must be addressed.

Treatment

Treatment of flexible pes cavus is from an orthotic device, which supports the plantar fascia by supporting the longitudinal arch, provides cushioning of the calcaneus, and protects the metatarsal heads. Any muscle imbalance must be ascertained and addressed with appropriate exercises.

HALLUS MALLEUS (HAMMER TOES)

History

Hallux malleus (hammer toes) refers to deformities of the toes with flexion contracture of the proximal interphalangeal joints combined with extension of the metatarsal joints. Calluses form on the tip of the flexed distal phalanx and at the dorsum of the flexed proximal interphalangeal joint.

Treatment

Determining the cause is important in advocating a treatment protocol, but the local condition, regardless of its cause, needs attention. Custom-made shoes called "space shoes" relieve the crowding of the toes and the pressure sites need appropriate padding. If there is failure, surgical intervention is suggested.[7]

REFERENCES

1. O'Donoghue DH. *Treatment of Injuries to Athletes*. 4th ed. Philadelphia, Pa: WB Saunders, Co; 1984.

2. Cailliet R. *Foot and Ankle Pain*. 3rd ed. Philadelphia, Pa: FA Davis Co; 1997.

3. Scranton PE Jr. Metatarsalgia: diagnosis and treatment. *J Bone Joint Surg Am*. 1980;62:723–732.

4. Stewart M. Miscellaneous affections of the foot. In: Edmonson AS, Crenshaw AH, eds. *Campbell's Operative Orthopedics*. 6th ed. St Louis, Mo: Mosby; 1980.

5. Inman VT, Ralston HJ, Todd F. *Human Walking*, Baltimore, Md: Williams & Wilkins; 1981.

6. Subotnik SI. The cavus foot. *Phys Sports*. 1980;8:53.

7. Turek SL. *Orthopedics: Principles and Their Application*. 3rd ed. Philadelphia, Pa: JB Lippincott; 1977.

chapter 8

Knee Impairment

The knee is a complex musculoligamentous structure with numerous tissues that respond to injury in specific ways. From an osseous structural viewpoint it is unstable without the support of the ligaments, menisci, capsule, and muscles (Figure 8.1).

TRAUMA

Trauma is the main source of impairment and may be external or internal. The incidence is described by the patient or visualized by an observer. The tissues affected by the trauma determines the resultant painful impairment.

External Injuries

External trauma are forces applied to the knee from any direction: anterior, lateral, medial, or in a rotatory manner. External injuries, as described by the patient or as visualized by an observer, are impact from the side or the front with the knee in various degrees of flexion or extension. The tissues that usually sustain the injury are the ligaments and possibly the menisci.

History
The patient recalls an injury and describes the physical force, the site of the injury, the force of the impact, and the resultant pain and immediate impairment. The extent of the pain, its intensity, and its relation to a specific movement is specified.

Diagnosis
The patient describes the pain and impairment and the physical examination verifies which tissues are injured and to what degree. Usually there is resultant joint fluid, which reveals deformation of

FIGURE 8.1

Knee Joint Viewed from front, knee complex includes these structures: tibia, femur, fibula, patella, medial meniscus (MM), lateral meniscus (LM), cruciate ligaments (CL), medial collateral ligament (MCL), and lateral collateral ligaments (LCL).

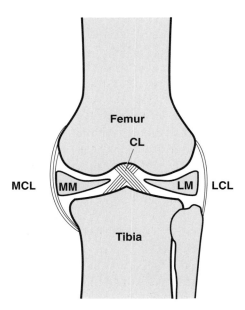

the joint and palpable edema. The presence of edema often makes a thorough evaluation of the limited range of motion impossible.

Aspiration of joint fluid is imperative as the discovery of a hemarthrosis (bloody fluid) indicates tearing and objective damage to the tissues within the joint. Removal of clear or cloudy fluid indicates inflammation but not specific tearing of joint tissues and permits a careful examination of the remaining tissues within the joint.

An external injury, such as force applied to the knee from the side or the front with the leg extended, causes disruption of the external ligaments. The medial and lateral ligaments are taut with the knee extended and relaxed as the knee flexes. This makes it important that the patient ascertains the knee position at the time of impact.

The history relates to the force experienced, and the resultant injury is noted in either the medial or lateral collateral ligaments. Local swelling and tenderness are noted. Further passive movement of the knee by the examiner causing either valgus or varus elicits pain and implicates the specific ligament injured. Passive valgus implicates the lateral collateral ligament; varus, the medial ligament.

Treatment

A clinical determination of a torn ligament requires a grading of its severity as its treatment will be influenced.

Grade I tears involve partial tears in the fibers of the ligament, but many fibers remain intact, affording stability. A lock knee brace for the first 4 to 5 days is followed by a hinged knee brace and exercises to strengthen the quadriceps, hamstring, and gastrocnemius muscles.

Immobilization must be followed by significant rehabilitation, as immobilization of the knee for a period as short as a week leads to marked atrophy of the quadriceps muscle group, which requires rehabilitation exercises for strengthening and endurance as well as proprioception balance training.[1]

Grade II injuries have nearly complete rupture of the ligament fibers but have an intact capsule. There is usually extensive swelling and hemorrhage. Initially the extremity is placed in a cast or brace flexed at 30 to 45 degrees of flexion for 1 week, then is replaced with a hinged brace allowing 10 to 90 degrees of motion. By the third week, the hinge permits 0- to 105-degree motion and, by the fourth week, full motion.

A grade III tear of the medial collateral ligament has tearing of the superficial and deep portions of the ligament, the surrounding portion of the capsule, and the oblique popliteal ligament. Surgical intervention is usually recommended.

Internal Injuries

Internal injuries to the structures of the knee do not implicate an external force or impact, but rather is an injury caused by specific movement of the patient.

History

An anterior or partially lateral external force can cause a translation or rotational injury injuring the cruciate ligaments. These ligaments restrict rotation and translation by their points of attachment and their course. The anterior cruciate ligament attaches from the anterior aspect of the tibia, then obliquely to the posterior aspect of the femoral head. By the oblique attachments they restrict excessive rotation and anterior-posterior translation.

The patient, having performed a sudden rotation upon the slightly flexed, weight-bearing knee, feels immediate pain, followed by a feeling of instability. Swelling occurs soon afterward and walking becomes impaired, as does flexing and re-extension of the weight-bearing knee.

Diagnosis

Clinically, the signs and symptoms of stress or tear of an anterior or posterior cruciate ligament are a feeling of instability, swelling, and pain. A thorough physical examination verifies that the cruciate ligament or ligaments have been elongated or torn.

The drawer test is performed with the patient placed in the supine position with the knee flexed to 90 degrees and the foot on the examining table and fixed there by the examiner. The lower leg is then passively translated (forward and backward) against the thigh (femur) and compared with a similar test of the uninjured leg. Excessive movement of the leg during translation will reveal ligamentous laxity or disruption of the anterior cruciate ligament if the leg moves further posteriorly, and disruption or tear of the posterior cruciate ligament if the leg moves further forward than normal. The presence and extent of a cruciate tear are determined with MRI.

Treatment

Management of a cruciate tear is either conservative exercises, as in the collateral ligaments, or surgical intervention if the tear is major or complete. A properly fitted brace reduces episodes of luxation and affords stability.

MENISCAL INJURIES

History

The menisci are cartilages that modify the congruity of the knee joint—the femoral condyles against the tibial plateaus.[2] The medial meniscus is attached to the collateral ligament and is injured much more frequently (80%) than the lateral meniscus, which is permitted freedom from the lateral collateral ligament.

The patient sustains an injury to the knee following a sudden rotational movement upon the weight-bearing knee. This is followed by swelling, local pain and tenderness, and difficulty in walking and climbing stairs.

Diagnosis

To confirm a damaged meniscus, the MacMurray test is performed. With the patient supine, the affected knee is fully flexed and gradually extended with simultaneous rotation. If there is painful grating and pain upon the maneuver, a tear in a meniscus is suspected. Grating at the beginning or the end of the flexion-extension indicates whether the tear is in the anterior or the posterior portion of the meniscus. Confirmation is obtained by computed tomography (CT) or magnetic resonance imaging (MRI).

Treatment

Tears in the meniscus occur at either end or as a circumferential (bucket) tear. If the tears do not permit the remaining meniscus to enter and impair joint motion, natural healing can occur. It is only where the remaining (untorn) meniscus impinges on the opposing surfaces of the tibial-femoral joint that surgical intervention is indicated.

PATELLOFEMORAL PAIN SYNDROMES

History

An irregularity called patellofemoral pain syndrome may develop in the cartilage of the patella. This knee impairment causes crepitation and pain during flexion-extension of the knee, especially when the quadriceps is strongly contracting, such as when the person is descending stairs.

Diagnosis

The patient identifies the site, and the history relates the action that produced the syndrome. The examiner can reproduce the symptoms by resisting or compressing the patella while having the patient contract the quadriceps muscle.

In attempting to determine the causative factors, the physician should consider the possibility of a weak quadriceps, weak hamstring muscles,[3] or abnormal femoral condyles causing abnormal patellofemoral contact.[4]

Treatment

Initially, relief of the acute inflammation is accomplished by rest, application of ice packs, and NSAIDs. If the pain and inflammation are severe, intra-articular injection of an analgesic agent and a steroid may help. Any physical weaknesses should be addressed by strengthening exercises. If there is a structural abnormality, a knee brace with a guiding patellar cutout may be of value.[5] Marked genu varus or vagus, which may cause improper tracking of the patellar alignment, must be addressed.

REFERENCES

1. Dillingham MF, King WD, Gamburd RS. Rehabilitation of the knee following anterior cruciate ligament and medial collateral ligament injuries. *Phys Med Rehabil Clin North Am.* February 1994;5:1.

2. Cailliet R. *Knee Pain and Disability.* 3rd ed. Philadelphia, Pa: FA Davis Co; 1992.

3. Radin EL. A rational approach to the treatment of patellofemoral pain. *Clin Orthop.* 1979;144:107–109.

4. Walla DJ, Albright JP, McAuley E, Martin RK, Eldridge V, El-Khoury G. Hamstring control and the unstable anterior cruciate ligament-deficient knee. *Am J Sports Med.* 1985;13:34–39.

5. Holden DI, Eggert AW, Butler JE. The nonoperative treatment of grade I and II medial collateral ligament injuries to the knee. *Am J Sports Med.* 1983;11:340–344.

Hip Impairment

Stress forces on the hip joint are massive. Compressive forces can be as high as 4 times the weight of the body.[1] The mechanical advantage of the hip joint occurs because the hip joint is the only true congruent joint in the body. Small deviations augment and localize the stress points of the joint, which move in all directions—flexion, extension, abduction, adduction, and rotation—mostly under compressive forces of the body weight and muscular contraction.

Cartilage coats most of the femoral head and the acetabular surface and is quite resilient. As in all cartilage, compression exudes fluid for lubrication and during relaxation (decompression) imbibes the joint fluid. At that phase, the joint fluid becomes nutrition for the cartilage.[2]

Total symmetry ensures longevity of the joint cartilage. It is possible, although not confirmed, that minor deviations of symmetry may cause alteration in cartilage metabolism with breakdown of structure.

Fracture of the hip joint or of the shaft or neck of the femur is a common source of impairment, especially among the elderly who have a degree of osteoporosis. These fractures, once discovered, heal well with wiring, pinning, rod insertion, or even with total hip replacement when severe. A repaired hip joint, with proper alignment, ensures good function and freedom from pain.

OSTEOARTHRITIS

Probably the most common cause of hip impairments is degenerative arthritis. This condition involves damage or destruction of the cartilage of the femoral head and ultimately of the acetabulum.

History

The etiology of degenerative arthritis remains obscure. There are 2 basic types of osteoarthritis. The first type is primary osteoarthritis, which is intrinsic disease of an otherwise normal joint. The other type is secondary osteoarthritis, which is a reaction to or sequel of a pre-existing condition, such as Legg-Calvé-Perthes disease (mentioned later in this chapter), or changes from a post traumatic fracture.[3] Familial predisposition has been reported, but minor mechanical abnormalities may have existed, such as variations in neck angle of inclination or angle of anteversion, that predisposed to ultimate cartilage degeneration (Figure 9.1).

Trauma to the surface integrity is the most commonly accepted precursor of osteoarthritis. Lubricants normally minimize friction resistance between bearing surfaces. Friction and wear between 2 irregular and unlubricated surfaces that glide on each other create rough surfaces that form osteoarthritic changes. (See Figure 1.7B in Chapter 1.)

Cartilage-on-cartilage lubrication depends on hyaluronic acid. A hyaluronate-free glycoprotein fraction has been isolated from synovial fluid that lubricates cartilaginous joints.[3]

In simple terms, cartilage functions just as an innerspring mattress functions with coils that resist compression (see Figures 1.9 and 1.10 in Chapter 1). Friction apparently shears the ends of the spring coils of the cartilage that decreases the compressive mechanical forces, which allow lubricant excretion and imbibition on relaxation.

Diagnosis

Clinically, the patient complains of pain while bearing weight on the affected side and of limited range of motion termed stiffness. In the early stages this stiffness will decrease as activity occurs, indicating that sufficient lubricant is still present and that there is sufficient cartilage remaining to separate the adjacent joint surfaces.

Occasionally, in the early changes, referred pain to the knee occurs, which confuses the examiner as to the precise site of impairment. This confusion is also accentuated when early radiologic studies fail to reveal changes in the joint space. In elderly patients the presence of osteoporosis with some minor stress fractures may also confuse the diagnosis.

FIGURE 9.1

Angles of Inclination and Anteversion A, Angle of inclination drawn from a line through neck (N) of femur (F) and through head of femur (H) and a line drawn through shaft of femur. Normal angle is 135 degrees. B, Angle of anteversion is angle formed by a line through neck (N) of femur (F) and a line drawn through condyles of tibia (TCA). Rotation of tibia (T) narrows the angle. A indicates acetabulum; H, head.

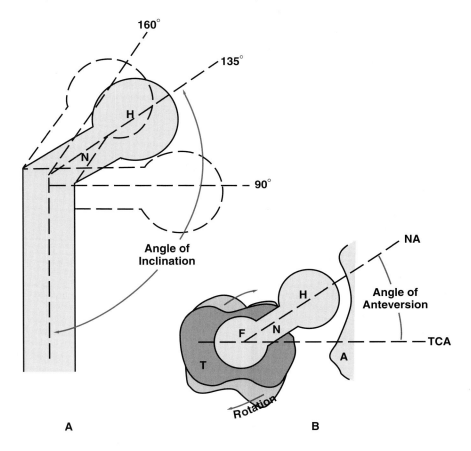

Treatment

Regardless of the cause, which cannot often be remedied, the condition demands attention in regard to pain and limitation of movement, which impairs ambulation and other activities of daily living. Medical management is benefited by use of oral salicylates, nonsteroidal anti-inflammatory drugs (NSAIDs), and intra-articular steroids. Weight loss is a valid treatment method, and the use of a cane in the opposite hand definitely diminishes weight bearing on the afflicted joint. It has been mathematically estimated that a cane in the opposite hand, held 20 inches from the center of gravity, decreases the weight born on the affected hip by 30%.[4]

Immobility or even limited range of motion is a risk factor for a joint contracture, which further limits motion of the joint and decreases the nutrition of cartilage with further deterioration.

Two factors limit joint range of motion.[5] One factor is arthrogenic restriction caused by bone, cartilage, synovium, capsule, and ligaments. The other factor is attributed to inflammation of muscle, tendon, and fascia. The former poses more problems in management, whereas the latter is more amenable to therapeutic intervention.

After intentional immobilization of a joint in one report in the literature,[5] the fixator was removed and the type of joint contracture was noted. Division of the contracted muscles allowed only a limited increased degree of motion, indicating that muscle tendon and capsule played only a minor role in joint contracture. The conclusion was that immobilization caused structural articular damage and the capsule contracture caused passive restriction. Whether the muscle component was shortened because of intrinsic nerve control (spindle cells and Golgi apparatus) was not confirmed.

In treatment of early degenerative disease of the hip joint, whether the resultant pain results from capsular, ligamentous contracture or cartilage erosion of joint surfaces or both, remains a moot point. With pain being addressed by numerous means, full range of motion must be maintained actively and passively, as this ensures adequate nutrition to the remaining cartilage. Full range of motion also ensures maintenance of adequate muscular strength.[6] Therapeutic ultrasound in conjunction with passive and active exercises has been shown to be effective in avoiding contracture. In exercises, the iliotibial band, hamstring muscles, hip flexors, and quadriceps and adductor muscles as well as the abductor and extensor muscles (gluteus maximus) must be stressed.[6,7]

LEGG-CALVÉ-PERTHES DISEASE

Legg-Calvé-Perthes disease in the young is a syndrome that is now considered to be ischemic necrosis of the head of the femur.

History

In a young child, before closure of the joint epiphysis, there occurs a limping due to pain first noted in the knee and then in the hip. Pain is only noted upon walking and then merely on weight bearing.

Limited motion occurs in which the child cannot flex or abduct the hip. The first symptoms are usually pain noted in the knee region and a limp after prolonged periods of walking, running, or jumping.

Diagnosis

The first findings are limited range of motion, especially external rotation and abduction of the hip. Initially, x-ray films may be negative but ultimately show evidence of necrosis with change in the contour of the femoral head. Early changes are noted in bone scans, which should be obtained when the syndrome is suspected.

Treatment

Treatment of Legg-Calvé-Perthes disease is to minimize weight bearing and maintain full range of motion of the hip. Use of a wheelchair and/or crutches in the acute stage is advocated, followed by the use of a cane. An ischial weight-bearing brace places the weight upon the ischium and on the joint. Exercises to maintain full range of motion and the strength of the hip muscles must be initiated and maintained until ossification is noted on radiologic studies.

REFERENCES

1. Andriacchi TP, Andersson GB, Fermier RW, Stern D, Galante JO. A study of lower limb mechanics during stair climbing. *J Bone Joint Surg.* 1980;62:749–757.
2. Chrisman OD. Biochemical aspects of degenerative joint disease. *Clin Orthop.* 1969;64:77–86.
3. Radin EL. Mechanical aspects of osteoarthritis. *Bull Rheum Dis.* 1976; 26:862–865.
4. Blount WP. Don't throw away the cane. *J Bone Joint Surg.* 1956;38A:695.
5. Trudel G, Uhthoff HK. Contracture secondary to immobility: is the restriction articular or muscular? An experimental longitudinal study in the rat knee. *Arch Phys Med Rehabil.* 2000;81:6–13.

6. Kaplan PE, Tanner ED. Hip joint dysfunction. In: Kaplan PE, Tanner ED, eds. *Musculoskeletal Pain and Disability*. Norwalk, Conn: Appleton & Lange; 1989.

7. Harris WH. Etiology of osteoarthritis of the hip. *Clin Orthop*. 1986; 213:20-33.

Somatic Pain Syndromes

Pain stemming from damaged tissues of the musculoskeletal system has been a major factor in the production of impairment and subsequent disability. A thorough discussion of musculoskeletal impairment cannot be considered without some discussion of the resultant pain. Important textbooks of medicine, surgery, and orthopedics rarely mention pain management.[1,2]

Pain was always described as a byproduct of a disease state—in orthopedics as an impaired musculoskeletal sequela of trauma or faulty function. The nociception products released or produced by trauma to any of the tissues irritate the end-organs of the sensory nerve supply of these tissues. The sensory nervous system was envisioned as merely a passive set of wires that transmitted electrical impulses to the brain. If the injured tissue was properly and promptly treated, the pain automatically subsided or disappeared.

This concept was prevalent before the writings of John Bonica[2] in the 1950s. In 1965, publication of the gate theory by Melzack and Wall[3] had a major impact on the concept of pain, in which the sensation was found to be modulated at the primary synapse and the brain. Primary transmission of the sensation from the site of tissue injury directly to the brain was refuted and further explored. The biopsychosocial approach became an integral part of pain management with modulation of afferent impulses. Merskey and Bogduk[4] wrote: "Pain is an unpleasant sensory and emotional experience associated with actual or potential tissue damage or described in terms of such damage."

CHRONIC PAIN

Chronic pain is a term implying prolongation of pain for more than 3 months despite natural recovery and accepted protocols of management. The neurobiology of chronic pain is currently unknown,

FIGURE 10.1

Somatosensory Pathways Terminating on Rexed Laminae in Dorsal Horn A beta fibers synapse on cells in laminae II and IV. A delta fiber synapse in cells in laminae I and V, and C fibers synapse in lamina II. After synapse, all of these fibers ascend spinal cord to thalamus. In small figure, SC indicates substantia gelatinosum; DH, dorsal horn.

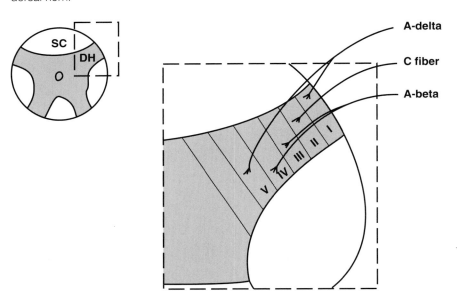

but current studies implicate chemical changes from the periphery centrally to the brain.

Chemical changes at the periphery in the musculoskeletal system act as nociceptors irritating nonmyelinated nerve endings of A alpha and C fibers. These chemical impulses ascend the nerve root to enter the gray matter of the spinal cord by passing through the dorsal root ganglion. Numerous chemicals are being identified almost daily (Figure 10.1).

It is at the spinal cord's dorsal horn (Rexed laminae I through V) that the gate theory of Melzack and Wall occurs (Figure 10.2).

Impulses originating from laminae I, II, and V cross the midline and ascend the spinothalamic tract of the spinal cord to ultimately synapse on thalamic nuclei (Figure 10.3).

FIGURE 10.2

Gate Concept of Melzack and Wall T cells located in lamina V transmit impulses to contralateral thalamus (T). These T cells are activated (+) from impulses from A beta, A delta, and C fibers. Impulses from substantia gelatinosum (SG) (Rexed laminae I and II) inhibit (-) T-cell impulses, as do impulses from C fibers. Inhibitory (–) impulses close the "gate," and facilitatory (+) impulses open the gate. L indicates large fibers; S, small fibers.

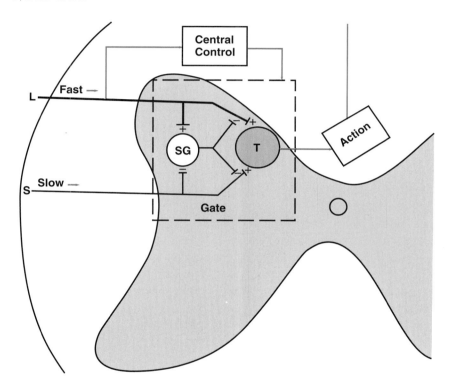

ACUTE PAIN

Acute pain results from the release of these nociceptor chemicals that are caused by trauma. Pain is usually of limited duration (48 to 72 hours) and responds to modalities such as ice, heat, and NSAIDs. An acute injury releases phospholipids, leading to leukotrienes and prostaglandin. Nonsteroidal anti-inflammatory drugs block this formation. The chemicals that form at the site of the tissue damage form what can be called nociceptive "soup" (Figure 10.4). This mixture includes, among others, glutamate, *N*-methyl-D-aspartate (NMDA), and substance P.

FIGURE 10.3

Transmission of Pain Trauma releases nociceptive chemicals that transmit to dorsal root ganglion cells (DRG), then to substantia gelatinosum (SG; Rexed layers I and II). Impulses then radiate to wide dynamic-range cells (WDR) and to lateral horn cells (LHC) that innervate sympathetic ganglia (SYM GGL), which supplies blood vessels (BV), hair follicles (HF), and sweat glands (SG). Synapse to anterior horn cells (AHC) is motor to peripheral muscles, which also contribute to reflex sympathetic dystrophy and paresis (see Chapter 11). LST indicates spinothalamic tract.

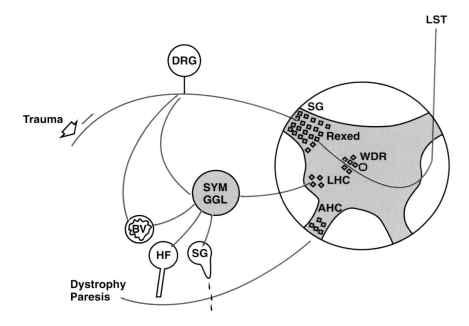

There are numerous nociceptive sites in the spinal cord from many musculoskeletal sites. (See Figure 2.14 in Chapter 2.)

Plasticity of the nervous system or learning has a role in pain. Repetitive noxious stimuli at the periphery are a source of continued pain, but it is clear that the brain can experience pain in the absence of peripheral stimulus. This has led to the postulation of *neuromatrix,* a concept of Melzack (Figure 10.5).

NEUROPATHIC AND NEUROGENIC PAIN

Pain arising from neuropathy remains hard to treat. The pathophysiology of neuropathic pain remains obscure, as most knowledge of neuropathic pain has been gained from animal studies, and animals cannot express pain except as withdrawal signs.

FIGURE 10.4

Inflammatory "Soup" for Pain Transmission "Soup" that forms and initiates impulses transmitted to dorsal root ganglion (DRG) along with nerve growth factors (NGF) ultimately synapses to dorsal horn neurons.

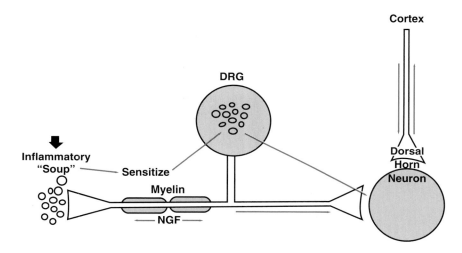

Neurogenic pain has been defined by the International Association for the Study of Pain as: "Pain initiated or caused by a primary lesion or dysfunction or transitory perturbation in the peripheral or central nervous system."[4] Neuropathic pain is a sub-entity in which there has been no "transitory perturbation." "Dysfunction" may also be a source of confusion because it allows nociception and psychogenic conditions to be improperly diagnosed as neurogenic or neuropathic.[5] Neurobiological impairment after a nerve injury can be considered as dysfunction, which makes the definition too broad. The diagnosis of neuropathic pain should be made only when the history and neurologic examination mandate that diagnosis.

PAIN AS A REACTION PATTERN

Gunn[6] specified that pain is a general reaction pattern: immediate, acute, and chronic. Immediate pain is a signal of tissue threat of damage mediated from nociceptors of inflammation (algesiogenic substance, such as histamine, bradykinin, and prostaglandin), transmitted via C and alpha fibers, hence "acute pain." Chronic pain may

FIGURE   10.5

Neuromatrix of Melzack Gate concept depicted in circle at left proceeds into neuro-matrix. SG indicates substantia gelatinosum; T, thalamus; and BG, basal ganglia.

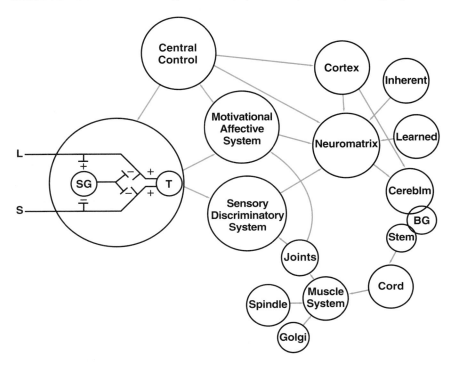

indicate ongoing nociception, functional structural alterations within the central nervous system, or psychological factors.

Patients suffering from neuropathic pain may have paroxysmal pain independent of a stimulus. This is termed *stimulus-independent pain* (Figure 10.6).

Fear of the trauma or the possibility of recurrence invokes further nociceptive activity that alters neural, hormonal, and behavioral reaction. (See Figure 2.16 in Chapter 2.)

In any trauma resulting in pain, there is noted migration (infiltration) of immune cells to the site of injury, such as perivascular macrophages, lymphocytes, and antigen-presenting cells. This infiltration evokes endothelial cells, microglia, and astrocytes to liberate cytokines and chemokines.[7,8] Glial cells (microglia, astrocytes, and oligodendroglia), which constitute more than 70% of the total cell population of the brain, were originally considered to be supportive tissues of neurons. These are now known to cause

FIGURE   10.6

Spontaneous Firing After Nerve Injury A, Trauma that injures the nerve evokes α-adrenoreceptors from nerve growth factors that are released from myelin sheaths. Neurons (DRN) of dorsal root ganglion (DRG) now become initiators of nociception. B, When stimulus has been severe and nerve axon is gone (dashed lines), dorsal root neurons (DRN) continue to fire without peripheral stimulus.

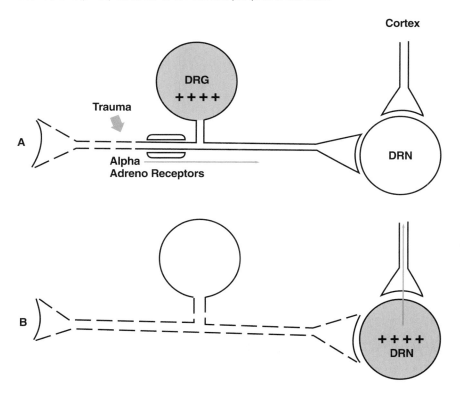

monocytes to release nociceptors, including cytokines and chemokines (Figure 10.7).

Cytokines are broadly classified as growth factors, interleukins, interferons, and tumor necrosis factors. They are synthesized locally at sites of inflammation and are distinct in the central nervous system. It has been found that physical training reduces the plasma levels of pro-inflammatory cytokines, which apparently explains why exercise is so valuable in treating fibromyalgia.

Acute pain is a chemical and psychological response to trauma that releases inflammatory chemicals at the nerve endings. Body healing mechanisms usually overcome these chemical reactions,

FIGURE 10.7

Release of Nociceptors from Injury to Glial Cells Trauma to glial cells, either mechanical or chemical, affect the monocytes of inflammation, which releases nociceptors.

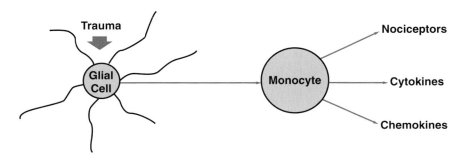

and intervention by pharmacologic or other modalities merely speeds the process of healing.

Chronic pain may result from ongoing nociception or inflammation, psychological factors, or neuropathic pain, which is associated with abnormal nerve function and/or hyperactivity at some level in the pain nervous system.

Gunn[9] postulates that chronic pain may occur because damage occurs to the nerves enclosed in the muscles that develop persistent contracture (spasm), and become hypersensitive from partial demyelination. He advocates early intervention by dry needling when these contracted muscles are discovered. In patients with chronic pain, a depletion of N-acetyl aspartate and glucose in the prefrontal cortex has been found. N-acetyl aspartate is located within neurons and is physiologically involved in the synaptic process. Breakdown of N-acetyl aspartate into aspartate becomes an excitatory amino acid neurotransmitter. This finding in chronic pain may lead to further discoveries of chemical depletions that may lead to therapeutic interventions.

REFERENCES

1. Loeser JD. Pain: an overview. *Lancet.* 1999;353:1607–1609.
2. Bonica JJ. *The Management of Pain.* Philadelphia, Pa: Lea & Febiger; 1953.
3. Melzack R, Wall PD. Pain mechanisms: a new theory. *Science.* 1965;150:971–979.
4. Merskey H, Bogduk N. *Classification of Chronic Pain.* Seattle, Wash: International Association for the Study of Pain Press; 1994.
5. Hansson P, Lacerenza M, Marchettini P. Aspects of clinical and experimental neuropathic pain: the clinical perspective. In: Hansson PT, Fields HL, Hill RG, Marchetini P, eds. *Neuropathic Pain: Pathophysiology and Treatment. Progress in Pain Research and Management.* Vol 12. Seattle, Wash: International Association for the Study of Pain Press; 2001.
6. Gunn CC, Sola AE. Chronic intractable benign pain (CIBP). *Pain.* 1989;39:364–365.
7. Sommer C. Cytokines and neuropathic pain. In: *Neuropathic Pain: Pathophysiology and Treatment. Progress in Pain Research and Management Series.* Vol 21. Hansson PT, Fields HL, Hill RG, Marchettini P, eds. Seattle, Wash: International Association for the Study of Pain Press; 2001.
8. DeLeo JA, Colburn RW, Nichols M, Malhotra A. Interleukin-6-mediated hyperalgesia/allodynia and increased spinal IL-6 expression in a rat mononeuropathy model. *J Interferon Cytokine Res.* 1996;16:695–700.
9. Gunn CC. *The Gunn Approach to the Treatment of Chronic Pain.* 2nd ed. New York, NY: Churchill Livingstone Inc; 1996.

Reflex Sympathetic Dystrophy (Complex Regional Pain Syndrome)

A diagnosis of reflex sympathetic dystrophy (RSD), more currently called complex regional pain syndrome (CRPS), continues to frustrate and perplex practitioners. When the diagnosis is not considered and addressed, affected patients are denied appropriate treatment.

The Committee for Classification of Chronic Pain of the International Association for the Study of Pain in 1994 provided standardized diagnostic criteria, albeit without specificity.[1] There are currently 4 salient diagnostic symptoms: (1) sensory (hyperesthesia), (2) vasomotor (temperature or skin color asymmetry or both), (3) sudomotor/edema (reports of asymmetrical edema in the affected limb and/or sweating asymmetry), and (4) motor/trophic (reports of motor dysfunction or trophic changes). Few if any objective signs are elicited, and there are no objective diagnostic procedures available in most clinics or offices.

HISTORY

Reflex sympathetic dystrophy was first described by Mitchell and coworkers[2] in 1964 as excruciating pain in an extremity after blunt (bullet) injuries suffered by soldiers in combat. None of the injured soldiers suffered a complete nerve disruption, but all had excruciating pain and hypersensitivity of the affected extremity that made even the touch of bed sheets or wind blowing from an open window unbearable. The description by Mitchell et al in its original language reads as follows:

In our early experience of nerve wounds, we met with a small number of men who were suffering from a pain which they described as "burning" or as "mustard red hot" or as "red hot file rasping the skin." The seat of the burning pain is very various but it never attacks the trunk, rarely the arm or thigh and not often the forearm or leg. Its favoured site is the foot or hand. In these parts it is found most often where the nutritive skin changes are met with. Its intensity varies from the most trivial burning to a state of torture which can hardly be credited, but which reacts on the whole economy until the general health is seriously affected. The part itself is not alone subject to intense burning sensation, but becomes exquisitely hyperesthetic, so as a touch or a tap of the finger increases the pain. Exposure to air is avoided by the patient with a care that seems absurd and most of the bad cases keep the hand constantly wet, finding relief in the moisture rather than the coolness of the application. As the pain increases, general sympathy becomes more marked. The temper changes and grows irritable and the face becomes anxious and has a look of weariness and suffering. The sleep is restless and the constitutional condition, reacting on the wounded limb, exacerbates the hyperesthetic states so that the rattling of a newspaper, a breath of air, a step of another across the ward, the vibrations caused by a military band, or shock of the feet in walking gives rise to increase of pain.

Three years later Mitchell used the word *causalgia,* which derives from the Greek words *kausis* (burning) and *algos* (pain). These symptoms were not originally termed *allodynia*, which is what current literature would use.

This painful condition was described before Mitchell by Sir James Paget[3] in 1864. He described an extremity as "glossy fingers which are usually tapering, smooth, hairless, almost devoid of wrinkles, pink, always associated with distressing and hardly manageable pain and disability."[3]

Fifty years after Mitchell's article, Leriche reported that sympathectomy dramatically relieved the causalgic pain. In 1967, Richards,[4] in an exhaustive review, described not only the clinical features but also the benefit from sympathetic blockade. The sweating, vascular abnormalities, and acute distal swelling (edema) of the affected limb often diminish after sympathetic blocks.[5]

The onset of the condition "without detectable nerve damage" was described early in the past century by Sudeck.[6] He claimed that the condition could occur from precipitating events such as fractures, soft-tissue injuries, strokes, myocardial infarcts, frostbites, and burns. He described onset of swelling and pain developing at a site distant from the tissue trauma. In 1946 Evans[7] called this syndrome "reflex sympathetic dystrophy."[8]

The relationship of the sympathetic nervous system to sensation and temperature regulation was first mentioned by Claude Bernard[9] in 1851, but its relationship to injury with resultant change of sensation and pain has been recognized only in the past 2 decades.

In 1986 Roberts[10] proposed the term *sympathetically maintained pain* as synonymous with RSD, because many patients with this syndrome responded to interruption of the sympathetic nervous system. However, because many patients suffering from nerve injuries and RSD sequelae did not respond to sympathetic intervention, the term, and the concept, of *sympathetically independent pain* was proposed. These 2 accepted yet differing syndromes exemplify the lack of diagnostic specificity of sympatholysis. No diagnostic tests have been proved specific for RSD or causalgia; thus, the diagnosis is based merely on clinical criteria. However, some tests and procedures are valuable tools that help confirm the clinical impression. Of these, the 3-phase bone scan indicates diffuse uptake of tracer around distal joints. Later radiographic studies reveal diffuse osteoporosis.

The classic criteria usually are:

1. A preceding noxious event with a nerve lesion or without a nerve lesion. Currently the former is termed CRPS type 1 and the latter is called CRPS type 2.
2. Spontaneous pain and hyperalgesia not limited to the expected dermatomic single-nerve territory.
3. Evidence or history of edema.
4. Skin blood flow (temperature) and sudomotor abnormality in the distal portion of the involved extremity.
5. Severity of symptoms out of proportion to the inciting event.
6. Other diagnoses excluded.

The syndrome occurs more often in females and affects the hands, feet, and knees most often. The event can occur after trauma, surgery, myocardial infarct, or brain infarct. In 5% of patients, no causes can be identified.[11]

Although there are no mechanisms currently accepted to explain the basis for this disorder, the role of the sympathetic nervous system is acknowledged because of the frequent benefit of the condition by interruption of the sympathetic nervous system.[12-14]

For almost a century, it has been assumed that activity in the sympathetic nervous system may be involved in the generation of pain. This assumption is based on the observation that the pain is spatially correlated with signs of autonomic dysfunction—abnormal blood flow, sweating, and trophic changes, as well as the pain being interrupted by blocking the efferent sympathetic nerve to the affected part.

Because of controversy over the involvement and cause of the sympathetic nervous system, a new taxonomy has evolved using the term *CRPS*, or *complex regional pain syndrome*. It is favored over RSD because the role of the sympathetic nervous system in many aspects of the illness is not clear and dystrophy may not occur in all patients.[11] The new term *CRPS* allows for later inclusions of painful syndromes after injury.

The Special Interest Group on Pain and the Sympathetic Nervous System of the International Association for the Study of Pain (IASP) developed a set of clinical descriptors to characterize features of the medical entities known as RSD and *causalgia*.[15] These studies led the IASP Subcommittee on Taxonomy to accept the term *CRPS*.

Complex regional pain syndrome has been arbitrarily divided into 2 types: CRPS 1 (RSD), the generic disease, and CRPS 2 (causalgia), a sequela of nerve damage. A third type, NOS (nitric oxide synthase), has been proposed for cases that do not fulfill the criteria of type 1 (Table 11.1) or type 2. Many patients suffering from the sequela of nerve injuries who do not respond to interruption of the sympathetic nervous system, yet have all the symptoms and signs of RSD, have the diagnosis of sympathetically maintained pain.[1] (Refer to Figure 10.3 in Chapter 10.)

More recently, diagnostic criteria made a distinction only between the 2 subtypes—CRPS 1 (RSD) and CRPS 2 (causalgia)—but noted that there should be subtypes so designated by their sequential stages.[16]

The early acute stage of CRPS (stage I) is characterized primarily by pain, sensory abnormalities such as hyperalgesia and allodynia (pain hypersensitivity to an otherwise innocuous stimulus), vasomotor dysfunction, edema, and sudomotor disturbances. Stage II, the dystrophic stage, occurs 3 to 6 months after onset and has greater and chronic pain and sensory abnormalities but marked motor and trophic changes. Stage III is the atrophic stage, with diminution of sensory symptoms but markedly increased motor or dystrophic tissue changes.

REGIONAL ANESTHESIA FOR DIAGNOSIS

The use of regional anesthesia for diagnosis of RSD (CRPS) has a long history that dates to World Wars I and II but has been reevaluated since the report of the IASP Subcommittee on Taxonomy when they

TABLE 11.1

IASP Diagnostic Criteria for CRPS 1*

1. Presence of an initiating noxious event, or cause of immobilization.
2. Continuing pain, allodynia, or hyperalgesia in which the pain is disproportionate to any inciting event.
3. Evidence at some time of edema, changes in skin blood flow, or abnormal sudomotor activity in the region of the pain.
4. The diagnosis is excluded by the existence of conditions that otherwise account for the degree of pain and dysfunction.

---

*IASP indicates International Association for the Study of Pain; CRPS 1, complex regional pain syndrome type 1.

changed the diagnostic label of RSD to CRPS 1 and CRPS 2. Before that, a diagnostic response to sympathetic blocks was considered needed to substantiate the diagnosis.

The response of sympathetically maintained pain (SMP) remains diagnostic in a negative way as sympathetic maintained pain does not need a positive response to sympathetic block for confirmation nor does CRPS.

Sympathetic blocks and sensory or motor nerve blocks remain pertinent diagnostically and therapeutically and need confirmation. Sympathetically maintained pain and sympathetically independent pain can and do coexist in many painful conditions, but only sympathetically independent pain reacts to sympathetic blocks.

The inflammatory component of CRPS types 1 and 2 has been well described, but their neurogenic component remains undetermined.[17] Early in the disease, when inflammation is most obvious, it is difficult to ascertain why pain relief can be produced by sympatholysis when, at this stage, postganglionic sympathetic activity is reduced.[18-20]

Intravenous regional block, using guanethidine and/or bretylium in addition to a local aesthetic agent, may be highly effective in the treatment of CRPS, although it cannot be used diagnostically. It may merely imply that the local anesthetic agent included in the intravenous regional block reduces or eliminates the inflammation affecting the involved vascular bed.

The technique of a stellate ganglion block has been well described in the literature.[21,22] Rather than at the classic injection site at the

C6 vertebra, the injection is probably best given at the C7 level. This approach allows the injected material to diffuse along the fascia of the musculus longus colli and to reach the T1 and T2 ganglia. With the use of larger amounts of local anesthetic (6 mL), it is possible to reach the T3 and T4 ganglia, ensuring more complete blocking of the upper extremity.

DENERVATION SUPERSENSITIVITY

Denervation supersensitivity was initially described by Cannon and Rosenblueth,[23] in what is now termed Cannon's Law. In a denervated tissue the law states:"when a series of efferent neurons in a unit is destroyed, an increased irritability to chemical agents develops in the isolated structures, the effects being maximum in the part directly innervated." Cannon and Rosenblueth showed that denervated striated muscle, smooth muscle, salivary glands, sudorific glands, autonomic ganglion cells, spinal neurons, and even central neurons within the cortex develop supersensitivity.

Actual physical interruption is not necessary for denervation super-sensitivity to develop; merely minor degrees of damage to motor neu-rons can result in supersensitivity from destruction of microtubules within the axon. These nerves still conduct nerve impulses and evoke muscular contraction, but the muscle cells innervated become super-sensitive as if the muscle had been totally denervated.[24-26]

Normally the area of receptivity in muscle is sharply circum-scribed to the end-plate region and occurs only at the synapse. After partial denervation, there is an increase in the surface area to sensi-tivity to acetylcholine, and changes occur at synapses.[27]

Denervation supersensitivity cannot completely account for the vasomotor and sudomotor abnormalities in CRPS, as there are often no overt nerve lesions and the autonomic symptoms spread beyond the territory of a lesioned nerve. Sweat glands do not develop dener-vation supersensitivity.[28] Therefore, the increased sweating in patients with CRPS probably relates to increased activity in the sym-pathetic nervous system and is of central origin.

A tendency to overdiagnose CRPS has been implied, as 37% of diabetic neuropathies fit the criteria of CRPS.[15] Although there are still many physicians who deny the existence of this syndrome, the preponderance of conferred diagnosis makes this syndrome a major disabling entity.

Complex regional pain syndrome is manifested predominantly in the distal extremities. However, in some cases it involves the trunk, face, or other sites as well as impairment of motor function, tremor, dystonia, and muscle weakness, hence the acceptance of the term *CRPS*. There is a temporal sequence as well as a regional aspect that justifies including all of these sites in the diagnostic label CRPS.

AUTONOMIC NERVOUS SYSTEM

Anatomically, the sympathetic nervous system is a highly complex arrangement of preganglionic and postganglionic neurons responsible for specific functions involving smooth, syncytial, and striated muscles.[29]

The manner of change, and how and why the sympathetic nervous system is involved in conditions without overt nerve damage, results in changes of blood flow, sweating, abnormal sensation, and dystrophy. The initial condition described by Mitchell and associates[2] in which a penetrating injury "adjacent to a major nerve gave rise to bizarre autonomic response of edema, heat, pain out of proportion to the injury, and allodynia" gives proof to this controversy.

Sympathetically maintained pain as a variant of CRPS or even as a nonpreexisting syndrome still creates a problem. Typical pain considered as RSD is blocked by α_1-blockers such as phentolamine and guanethidine. However, as the disease progresses and becomes chronic, the pain changes from sympathetically maintained pain to sympathetically independent pain. Sympathetically maintained pain is characterized by upregulation and supersensitivity to norepinephrine. α-Adrenoceptor agonists either injected or applied by iontophoresis to an extremity previously affected but in remission for 10 to 15 years would develop symptoms of CRPS[30-35] (Figure 11.1).

A continuous functional inhibition of vasoconstrictive activity induced by central mechanisms may lead to secondary end-organ supersensitivity in the absence of structural damage to the sympathetic fibers.[28] The clinical picture changes from the concept of inflammation to neuropathic pain.

Intravenous injections of phentolamine in patients considered as having sympathetically maintained pain showed no difference in benefit compared with placebo controls; thus, the diagnosis of sympathetically maintained pain was questioned (Figure 11.2).

There are clinical variants of RSD, as shown below:[36]

Causalgia	RSD symptom complex occurring after a peripheral nerve injury
Minor causalgia	RSD symptoms with predominant hypalgesia with no nerve injury
Major causalgia	RSD occurring after a peripheral nerve injury

FIGURE 11.1

Sympathetic Impulses Trauma enters spinal cord gray matter (SG) through dorsal root ganglion (DRG) to wide dynamic-range nuclei (WDR) and synapses with lateral horn cells (LHC), progressing to sympathetic ganglia (SYM GGL). Sympathetic efferent impulses discharge norepinephrine into vesicles that stimulate α_1-receptors.

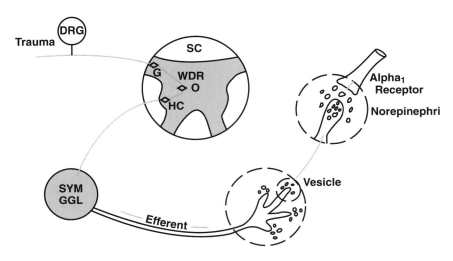

Mimo-causalgia	RSD symptom complex, which occurs after insult to the CNS
Sudeck atrophy of bone	RSD symptom complex, which occurs after soft-tissue injury with bone atrophy as a predominant finding
Shoulder-hand syndrome	RSD syndrome complex with "frozen shoulder" occurring after myocardial infarction, cerebro-vascular accident, or cervical radiculopathy

STAGES OF CRPS

Clinically, CRPS in its early stages demonstrates pain more severe than expected from the trauma or other cause. The characteristic pain spreads progressively in regional distribution and is not dermatomic. The pain is characteristically described as "burning" from its onset and is both superficial and deep. The pain is accompanied by hyperalgesia of greater intensity than is expected from stimulus and allodynia. Gradually, if not rapidly, there occurs hyperpathia (an increased threshold to pain that, when exceeded, reaches maximal intensity too quickly and is not bound to the intensity of the stimulus).

FIGURE 11.2

Formation of Sympathetic Nervous System Typical nerve root with sympathetic fibers. Somatic nerves (DR) pass through dorsal root ganglion (DRG) to form visceral efferent nerve (VE). Sympathetic nerve originates at lateral horn cells through ventral root (VR), merges with somatic fibers, and enters paravertebral ganglion (PVG) through gray ramus communicans (GRC); it then emerges via white ramus communicans (WRC).

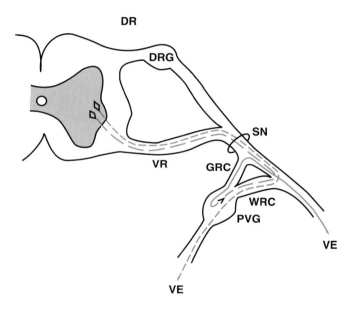

Other than pain, there occur signs of vasomotor instability, with the involved extremity becoming cold (or hot), moist (hyperhidrosis), dusky colored (cyanosis), and progressively edematous. Signs of vasomotor instability may not be present at the time of clinical examination but are described by the patient and are important in making the diagnosis.

In stage II, the edematous tissue becomes indurated, and the skin is cool and hyperhidrotic with some cyanosis. Some hair loss occurs, and the nails show ridging. Pain is constant as well as characteristic, and allodynia is prevalent. Bone scanning becomes diagnostic, and some osteoporosis is seen on radiologic studies.

In stage III, characteristic pain spreads proximally but in a nondermatomic area.

There is growing evidence that oxygen metabolism is impaired in CRPS. Muscle biopsy specimens from amputees with incurable CRPS show hypoxic changes in blood vessels and muscle fibers similar to those found in diabetic individuals with proven impairment of microcirculation.[37]

It is known that tissue acidosis is a regular finding in ischemia and inflammation.[38] Experimental tissue acidosis caused pain in the affected limb similar to that experienced in CRPS, raising the question whether tissue acidosis contributes greatly to the pathophysiology of CRPS. Venous lactate concentrations are increased in the CRPS-affected limbs, probably caused by perfusion abnormalities in CRPS because of central sympathetic dysfunction.

DIFFERENTIAL DIAGNOSIS

There are many conditions with characteristics of CRPS that must be ruled out:

- diabetic neuropathy,
- arachnoiditis,
- nerve root contusion,
- nutritional neuropathy,
- vasculitis, and
- multiple sclerosis.

Among these conditions also include the following, which may lead to CRPS:

- cumulative trauma disorder,
- repetitive strain syndromes,
- overuse syndrome,
- shoulder-hand syndrome,
- fibromyalgia, and
- peripheral vascular disease.

MECHANISMS OF REFLEX SYMPATHETIC DYSTROPHY

Leriche[5] first postulated that the etiology of RSD was a dysfunction of the sympathetic nervous system (Figure 11.3) when he relieved symptoms by denervating the blood vessels of their autonomic nerves (Figures 11.4, 11.5).

FIGURE 11.3

Autonomic Sympathetic Nervous System Autonomic sympathetic nervous system (SYM) runs parallel to somatic nervous system (BVC) and innervates heart (H) and blood vessels (BV) from ganglia.

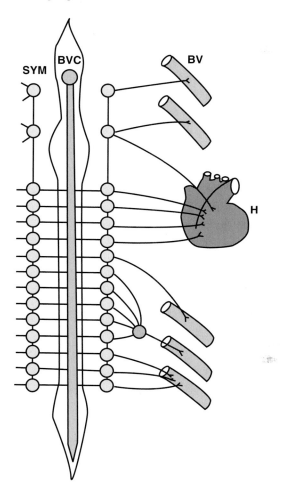

Denervation, surgically or chemically, does not always relieve the symptoms of CRPS. More recent research has emphasized the supersensitivity of the sensory α-adrenoreceptors rather than efferent sympathetic nerves as the causative factor. This is a contradictory statement, in a way, as both are directly related to the sympathetic nervous system.

FIGURE **11.4**

Innervation of Blood Vessels Sensory afferent fibers (S) enter dorsal horn substantia gelatinosum (SG; Rexed laminae I and II) via dorsal root ganglia (DRG), then connect to lateral horn cells (LHC) and then to blood vessel. There is also synapse to anterior horn cell (AHC) that innervates muscles. SYM indicates sympathetic; STT, spinal thalamic tract; and M, motor.

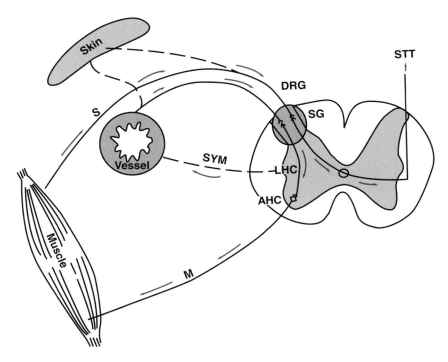

The autonomic nervous system (ANS) is divided into 2 systems—sympathetic and parasympathetic—which normally remain in balance.

The sympathetic nervous system has 3 major physiological roles: regulation of body temperature; regulation of vital signs, which include blood pressure, pulse rate, and respiration; and regulation of the immune system. These 3 functions protect the internal environment of the body. These functions are mediated by afferent sensory mechanisms (thermoreceptors, mechanoreceptors, and chemoreceptors); efferent vasomotor responders (control of the immune system); and modulation of the limbic nervous system controlling the emotions. All are involved and essentially affected in CRPS.

FIGURE 11.5

Typical Arterial Blood Vessel Typical blood vessel is shown that contains red blood cells within lumen, which is controlled by arterial muscles that are under control of sympathetic nervous system (ANS).

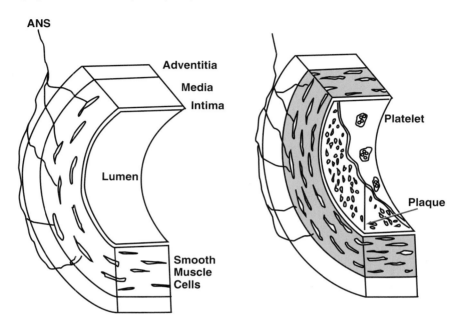

The types of pain involved in CRPS are transmitted through various types of nerves: hyperpathia (pain) via nonmyelinated nerves (C thermoreceptors); allodynia via myelinated A beta nerve fibers; and causalgia (burning pain) via nonmyelinated chemoreceptors.

Hyperpathia, also termed *protopathia*, is intense persistent "burning quality" pain. In CRPS it is usually out of proportion to the severity of the inciting trauma. It varies from being constant (75%) to intermittent (25%).[39] Simple tactile stimulation of the area described as the affected area may be accompanied by an objective rise in pulse rate and blood pressure, indicating the sympathetic component of RSD pain.

Because thermal regulation is a function of the sympathetic nervous system, the innervation is to blood vessels and sweat glands. This explains why the pain pattern is thermatomic and not dermatomic, as in somatic nerve distribution (Figure 11.6).

FIGURE 11.6

Dermatomes of Upper Extremity Dermatomes of nerve roots of cervical spine from C4 to T1.

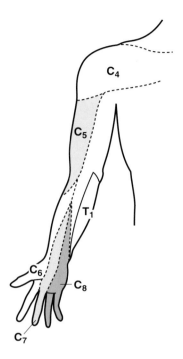

The thermatomic patterns are in the distribution of the brachial, femoral, carotid or mesenteric arteries. Spread of pain, which is a factor in making the diagnosis of CRPS, is the result of summation of repetitive stimulation of the thermoreceptors. The spread patterns are horizontal or vertical and may even be to the opposite side (Figure 11.7).

Hyperpathic pain is predominantly activated by the thermal C nociceptive sensory fibers. Afferent small C-fiber systems may be inhibited by larger A-fiber myelinated somatosensory fibers. When these small C fibers are lost due to hypersensitivity, the inhibitory factor is lost. There results increased firing of the afferent pain fibers and increased sensitivity of the Rexed laminae I and II.[39]

The distribution of allodynia is not in the distribution of somatic nerves. Mechanical allodynia is mediated by A beta, low-threshold, small myelinated mechanoreceptor nerves.

FIGURE 11.7

Spread Patterns of Pain A, Posterior view of areas of spread of pain—hyperpathia and allodynia—in upper extremity. B, Anterior view. Only upper extremity is shown, but there are similar patterns in lower extremity.

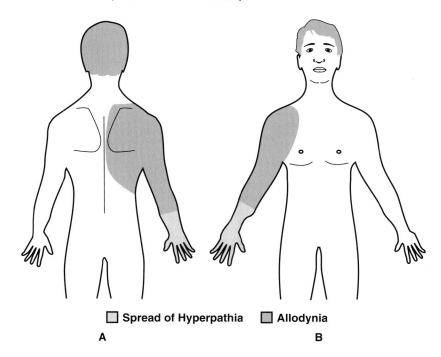

☐ **Spread of Hyperpathia**   ▨ **Allodynia**
A   **B**

As depicted by infrared thermal imaging, there is a central hyperthermia surrounded by a margin of hypothermia. Application of ice, often proposed as a treatment, exaggerates vasoconstriction, causing nerve damage with greater allodynia and actually causing sympathetically maintained pain to become sympathetically independent pain.

Currently considered mostly a peripheral nerve affliction, CRPS is a "complex neurological disease involving various levels of integration of the brain."[40] Under normal conditions, activation of the sympathetic nervous supply to somatic tissues does not generate pain, but in patients with CRPS 1 and CRPS 2, pain resulted in the extremities being maintained at a constant temperature of 35°C. Cooling the body, which enhances activity in cutaneous vasoconstrictor neurons, indicates that the pain was not predominantly due to vasoconstriction, because the extremity vessels did not constrict.

This finding confirms the generation of pain from sympathetic activity but does not explain its mechanism. In CRPS types 1 and 2, there is sensitization and persistent activity of intact primary afferent neurons (mostly C fibers); therefore, there must be "central sensitization."[40]

Complex regional pain syndrome type 1 is more common than CRPS 2, which occurs without a nerve lesion, yet is "neurologic" because it occurs after trauma without a detectable nerve lesion and may involve deep somatic tissues. Its mechanism must consider dynamic long-term "central" changes. These changes imply changes in central representations in the spinal cord, brain stem, thalamus, and forebrain, albeit that the primary lesion is peripheral.

These central changes may be irreversible, and it is well accepted that there are no detectable changes in the peripheral nerves. A "positive feedback" has been proposed by Janig et al.[39,41,42]

Causalgic pain described as "lightning" or "electric shock" is often accompanied by myoclonus (jerks of the muscles) of the extremity. This is considered to be due to the damaged myelinated (sensory) nerve stimulating adjacent partially damaged (motor) nerves. These impulses are blocked by phentolamine sympathetic blocks given in the early stages of CRPS.[40]

It is recognized that inactivity is a detrimental factor in prolonging or aggravating the deep pain symptoms of CRPS and is to be avoided. Inactivity causes a chemical reactivity of the deep chemoreceptor nerves within muscles and bone. It is considered to be the cause of pain upon awakening in the morning after a period of inactivity. It is also a basis for enforced activity in the treatment protocol.

Disuse is rarely addressed in scientific articles, yet encouraging patients with CRPS to become active is advocated as mandatory in all treatment protocols. Symptoms similar to CRPS have been noted after prolonged cast immobilizations of extremities.[43]

After immobilization, patients show involvement of the brain centers associated with sensory processing, pain, and motor function. These findings indicate that long-standing pain with consequent immobilization can cause central changes in the central nervous system (CNS) from the dorsal horn of the cord centrally. These central changes are noted in CRPS 1 and may indicate why management of this syndrome has so many failures.

Prolonged immobilization from any basis causes muscle atrophy; joint stiffness; skin discoloration; and often thickness of the skin, hair, and fingernails. These findings are explained by vasomotor changes and are expected and usually short-lived and reversible. Only when prolonged and accompanied by characteristic pain, allodynia, and hypersensitivity is the diagnosis of CRPS 1 considered.

Researchers at the University of Washington Pain Center have long believed that immobility alone is responsible for most of the signs and symptoms of CRPS 1, because during casting an increase in cerebral blood flow in areas of sensory perception are noted in positron emission tomographic (PET) studies.[44]

Early intervention, both active and passive, of an involved extremity reverses the CNS changes noted after immobilization. Pain can be produced by immobilization alone.[44-46]

Pain after total knee replacement occurs frequently and is hard to explain, as all the tissues that caused the pain before surgery are removed. Many of these "unexplained pains," described as "aching," "throbbing," and "sharp," are considered CRPS 1.[47]

Movement disorder, tremor, spasms, and dystonia, so frequently experienced by patients with RSD, are considered to be due to enlargement of the central pain projecting neurons in Rexed laminae I and II of the spinal cord. These layers respond to discharge of C nociceptor and A alpha fibers, whereas laminae IV and V exert inhibitory function on laminae I and II. Chronic repetitive release of neuropeptide chemicals (calcitonin gene-related peptide [CGRP], substance P, and nitric acid) hypersensitize the laminae I and II and diminish the inhibitory effects of laminae IV and V.

Movement disorders of CRPS may be a manifestation of deafferentation and sensitization of the spinal cord due to long-term afferent damage to the inhibitory granular cells in laminae I and II. These movements appear in later stages of the disease process.

Impaired integration of visual and sensory afferent inputs to the parietal cortex has been implicated as the basis of motor deficits in patients with CRPS.[48]

Rarely, both arms and legs are affected. In dystonia of the upper extremity, the dystonia begins with flexion contracture of the fourth and fifth fingers of the affected hand. It evolves into adduction and flexion of the arm and wrist. These manifestations may be alleviated by sympathetic blockade if given early.

Emotional aspects of CRPS are based on the direct effect on the limbic system. Compared with somatic sensory fibers, the sensory neuropathic fibers (90%) terminate in the limbic system.

LABORATORY DIAGNOSTIC TESTS

The ANS is an extensive neural network that controls homeostasis and visceral functions. Most ANS functions are out of conscious control, but emotions and somatosensory inputs profoundly influence the ANS. Its specific role in mediating and transmitting pain remains unanswered.

The ANS has both a central and peripheral component. The central component includes the insula, medial prefrontal cortex, hypothalamus, amygdala, ventrolateral medulla, nucleus of the tractus solitarius medullae oblongatae, nuclei parabrachiales, periaquaductal gray matter, and circumventricular organs.

The insula is the crucial area with its connection with the hypothalamus, which is the most important organ of the ANS controlling the endocrine and autonomic systems. The periductal periaquaductal gray matter is a crucial structure in pain modulation.

The peripheral components of the ANS include the sympathetic system, in which the preganglionic neurons lie in the intermediolateral columns of the spinal cord and their axons synapse in the prevertebral and paravertebral ganglia. The sympathetic system generates epinephrine release from the adrenal medulla via its postganglionic fibers. Acetylcholine is the neurotransmitter in both preganglionic and postganglionic fibers at their synapses.

There are no specific tests that confirm the diagnosis, but certain diagnostic tests may add a rational approach to management of the syndrome.

Skin temperature and cutaneous blood flow show abnormalities in the distal part of the extremity affected by CRPS, and thermoregulatory reflexes to whole-body heating and cooling are also abnormal.[49] Tests include thermometry, telethermometry, and thermography.[50,51]

A major consequence of sympathetic failure in CRPS is loss of blood flow control in the affected limb with loss of microcirculation control; this leads to arteriovenous precapillary blood shunting, which, because of the malnutrition to the skin, results in dystrophic changes.[52,53] Peripheral blood flow can be measured by Doppler flowmetry and quantitative sudomotor axon reflex tests.[54] The quantitative sudomotor axon reflex test (QSART) requires equipment consisting of a 3-compartment capsule, a constant flow of nitrogen (N_2) to evaporate the sweat, and a heat exchanger to detect the thermic change due to moisture of the returning N_2 flow. A solution of 10% acetylcholine is injected into the first compartment, and a constant current of 2 mA is applied for 5 minutes. Sweat output is measured for 5 minutes after the stimulus is discontinued. After a stable baseline is obtained, 4 sites are tested simultaneously: medial distal aspect of the forearm, proximal lateral aspect of the leg, medial distal aspect of the leg, and dorsum of the foot.

In the thermoregulatory sweat test (TST), the patient disrobes and is dusted with alizarin red powder. When moist, the powder changes color from orange to purple. A thermal probe is placed in the patient's mouth and another on the skin. The patient enters a closed compartment heated by infrared heating units that control humidity and ambient temperature. The patient is then heated to a core temperature 1°C above baseline. If profuse sweating occurs, the test is stopped and the patient is photographed. Computer scans of the areas are then mapped, and the patterns of hypohidrosis and anhidrosis are evaluated.[55-57]

Manual muscle strength testing is the most available diagnostic test in CRPS and determines the patient's pain threshold and compliance and cooperation. Joint range of motion is also tested.

Psychological testing using the Beck Depression Inventory or the McGill Pain Questionnaire is valuable for projecting the patient's perception of the disease and the indication for intervention.

TREATMENT INTERVENTIONS

Numerous treatment protocols have been advocated in the management of CRPS. Some or all are effective in some cases, but not all have been evaluated in a double-blind manner consistent with Cochran protocols. In addition, they do not specifically address the goals of RSD, in which the dystrophic changes, and not merely pain, are the biggest challenge.

Guidelines for treatment were well standardized by Stanton-Hicks et al.[14,58] The authors stated that the condition being treated must fit the IASP's revised description, which must have clinical symptoms that include pain, sensory changes such as allodynia, abnormalities of temperature, abnormal sudomotor activities, edema, and an abnormal skin color.[15] All of these symptoms and findings must be addressed in any treatment protocol and in a preferential sequence.

The algorithm proposed by the specialists quoted by Stanton-Hicks et al[58] was in 4 phases, with early intervention being mandatory. The first phase consisted of influencing behavior and getting patient rapport by a clear understanding of the problem and its solutions. The second phase was addressing pain that could intervene in the needed rehabilitation process to follow. The third phase involved modalities that diminished the dystrophic phase of the condition, and the fourth phase was a return to normal daily functions. Each phase advocated was formulated to occur within 2 or 3 weeks to be effective; if the phase was prolonged, the patient was given psychotherapeutic intervention and more aggressive management

After initial discussion of the condition and assurance of patient compliance, pain must be addressed to ensure further compliance. Painful neuropathies may accompany any lesion of the peripheral or central nervous system in which all neuropathic pains project to the innervation area of the damaged nerve. Painful neuropathies are characterized by spontaneous and/or stimulus-evoked pain. The "allodynia" described by Mersky and Bogduk,[1] as mentioned, is pain evoked by a usually innocuous stimulus, whereas hyperalgesia is pain evoked by a normally painful stimulus. This allodynia or hypersensitivity to pain present the greatest challenge to application of most other modalities.

As sympathetic dysfunction is assumed in the etiology of CRPS, it must be addressed early. Despite support from animal experiments, proof of the effectiveness of sympathetic blockade for the treatment of CRPS remains scanty, but sympathetic blockade warrants use in management.

There are 3 basic techniques for administration of sympathetic blockade: (1) surgical sympathectomy, (2) local anesthetic injection around the sympathetic ganglia of the affected part, or (3) regional intravenous application of guanethidine, bretylium, or reserpine. Intravenous injection of phentolamine is used to diagnose sympathetically dependent pain. It must be remembered that not all conditions considered as sympathetically initiated and maintained are ameliorated by interruption of the sympathetic nervous system.

If the first block is initially effective, any later recurrence or persistence of symptoms may indicate the need for a repeated block. Its efficacy must be evaluated by the presence of a Horner syndrome, indicating that sympatholysis has occurred. An increase in the temperature of the fingers must also have occurred.

Continuous conduction blocks of the brachial or lumbar plexus may be used for periods of 6 weeks. Epidural injections of analgesic and steroids are also of value and again can be administered for prolonged use by insertion of an epidural catheter.

Phentolamine infusion may be as effective as stellate blocks, but whichever succeeds in decreasing the allodynia and "burning pain" hyperalgesia should be used. Once there is evidence of efficacy, further modalities to improve function will be easier to institute.

Because early CRPS usually has evidence of inflammation, rubor, edema, and heat, the use of steroids is considered valid especially if sympathetic blocks are not totally or acceptably effective. Oral corticosteroids are also valuable. A trial of corticosteroids is warranted if sympathetic blockade relieves spontaneous pain, but the clinician of today uses a course of steroids early in any suspected case of CRPS and often with some benefit.

Stanton-Hicks et al,[58] in their proposed algorithm, imply that restoration of function is the primary goal of treatment, with which all therapists can agree. They also claim that "medications, analgesics including regional anesthesia, neuromodulation and psychotherapy are only agents designed to facilitate this restoration of function."

In functional restoration, mobilization can be accomplished only by desensitization of the involved tissues. Desensitization is attempted by medications that reduce pain and the simultaneous use of modalities that desensitize the tissues to allow movement and decrease tactile sensitivity.[58,59]

Kinesiophobia must be allayed early by impressing on the patient that pain from movement is not synonymous with damage. It must be explained to the patient why any movement may be painful but that to allow pain to govern return of range of motion, and thus function, must be avoided. Sensitivity to touch must also be explained, and its occurrence must be accepted.

The pain of CRPS may be spontaneous, aching, and deep in perception and may be aggravated by touch, thermal stimulation, or orthostasis (dependency of the involved extremity). All or any of these must be considered in determining both the modality prescribed in the treatment protocol and the efficacy of that treatment.

Physical Therapy

Cryotherapy is often used in decreasing hypersensitivity and allodynia of the involved extremity. Application of ice (cryotherapy) to the inflamed part may be used to reduce the local heat of the tissue, lessen abnormal muscle tone, relieve pain by raising the threshold of pain receptors, and lessen local circulation to diminish the formation of edema.[60]

Temperatures (cooling) that affect spasticity do not affect sensory feedback, so they do not affect skill training. Cooling may affect gamma fibers, but the sensitivity of these fibers is less than that of the spindle fibers. With prolonged cooling, there is a decline in muscle tone and in reflexes.[61]

Bell and Lehmann[61] measured skin and muscle temperatures before and after cold applications. They found that there was a decrease of skin temperature to 18.5°C (65.3°F) and of the muscle temperature to 12.0°C (53.6°F), with a decrease also in the M reflex. Therefore, after application of cold, both muscle temperature and motor tone are decreased. Sensory nerve fibers also lose sensitivity, as was found by Melzack and Wall.[62]

Review of the literature on the effects of heat or cold reveals a similar effect from both.[63] Pain may be reduced from both cold and heat, but heat increases blood flow and cold decreases it. Edema is increased with heat and decreased with cold. Tolerance is therefore important as to whether the patient can tolerate either with the presence of allodynia or hypersensitivity. Temporal factors must also be taken into consideration as to how long either should be applied. Joint stiffness is decreased with heat and increased with cold, and prolonged application of cold can impair nerve function.

A recent publication demonstrated that in sympathetic maintained pain syndrome, physiological activation of cutaneous vasoconstrictive neurons projecting to the painful arm or leg enhances spontaneous pain and hyperalgesia.[63] The authors thus postulated a pathological interaction between sympathetic and afferent neurons within the skin.

Peripheral nerve damage (in CRPS type 2 and sympathetically maintained pain) induces a functional change in the phenotype of primary C-nociceptor neurons. These neurons start to express adrenoceptors at their membranes, which become sensitive to sympathetic trunk stimulation.

This stimulation was enhanced by a unique technique.[64] Microneurographic recordings of skin nerves revealed vasoconstriction inhibition on whole-body warming and activated on whole-body cooling. This whole-body cooling and warming was accomplished by application of the patient in a thermal suit in which circulating water of 12°C or 50°C was used to cool the entire body. The suit did not cover the arms or legs, which were tested by laser Doppler instruments, applied to the fingers or toes, and by infrared thermography. Pain intensity was coded as expressed by the patient.

To overcome barriers of movement and articular limitation, exercises should be initiated early. It remains controversial as to whether limited joint disease is originally neuromuscular from sustained muscular contraction or intrinsic disease from gravity.

Exercises

Isometric contraction of muscles usually will be tolerated in the early stage of CRPS. *Isometric* implies contraction of muscle without movement of the joint, which is often painless and gives sensory feedback of the action; not moving the joint causes little pain and kinesiophobia to the patient. Whether isometric contraction of muscle is done actively or by electrical stimulation to the muscles is a matter of judgment by the therapist and acceptance by the patient. Ultimately, isotonic exercises must be initiated, as this type of exercise causes hypertrophy of the muscles, increases endurance and strength, and physiologically moves the joint.

Increased range of motion of the joint or joints to physiological range is the goal of therapy, as only by reaching this goal can total function be restored. The restoration of range of motion can be initiated passively but requires diminishing allodynia, hypersensitivity, and muscular contraction. It also demands a cognitive behavior approach to pain avoidance techniques such as overprotection and movement phobia by voluntary bracing.

Severe cutaneous allodynia can prevent appropriate treatment by any modality that requires the part being touched. Allodynia can be diminished, if not eliminated, by the application of ice and heat and by the use of massage, brushing, or scrubbing.

All these modalities may require the use of regional anesthesia and even the use of general anesthesia. Nerve block of the nerve supply to the affected body part, performed with lidocaine or even longer-acting bupivacaine hydrochloride (Marcaine), will permit beneficial local modalities to be used.

Paravertebral blocks are also beneficial. While the body part is anesthetized, gentle mobilization or manipulation of the affected joint can also be performed. If the increased range of motion remains unacceptable to the patient, a cast may be applied to the affected joint to maintain that gained range. The cast may be bivalved to permit the part to be removed and locally treated; then the cast can be replaced. A dynamic cast may be applied that incorporates a hinge to progressively increase the range.

Edema must be aggressively approached by compressive dressing, elevation of the swollen body part, and even dynamic compression by a sleeve unit. Edema in a finger or fingers can be reduced by use of a twine wrapped from distal to proximal aspects, with increasing compression.

Topical application of transdermal lidocaine has been proved effective. Topical capsaicin, proved effective in other neuropathies, has merit in use for patients with CRPS.

Pharmaceutical Management

Numerous medications have been used in the treatment of CRPS, but none has yet been accepted as the unequivocal standard or as predictably effective. Those listed here are currently considered effective.

Nonsteroidal anti-inflammatory drugs (NSAIDs) that inhibit cyclooxygenase are considered beneficially algesic and can be used early in the management of CRPS. They must be properly prescribed as to dosage and possible side effects.

Opioids usually are considered ineffectual in neuropathic pain but, as their efficacy varies with individual cases, they merit trial. The patient should be fully informed of the possibility of addiction and other undesirable effects.

Tricyclic antidepressants have been considered a primary beneficial medication for management of neuropathic pain,[65-67] as was discussed earlier in this text. Besides decreasing pain and hypersensitivity, they act in treating depression and anxiety, which often exist in prolonged recalcitrant cases of CRPS. These drugs also improve sleep, which is often impaired.

As also mentioned previously, anticonvulsants (membrane stabilizers) and α-blockers (eg, terazosin, phenoxybenzamine) have been proved effective in treating neuropathic pain, but their undesirable side effects make their use questionable. Additionally, propranolol has also been claimed effective, as has γ-aminobutyric acid (GABA). Recently the German drug mexiletine, which is an oral antiarrhythmic lidocaine analogue, has been found effective in diabetic neuropathy. By the time of this publication, many other drugs will have been proposed and will be awaiting clinical testing.

Of great value are Bier blocks using lidocaine and corticosteroids with reserpine or guanethidine, which accumulate the medications distal to the tourniquet and thus enhance their efficacy locally in the extremity.

Transcutaneous electric nerve stimulation has its advocates and merits. When CRPS becomes resistant to conservative conventional therapeutic measures and remains totally impairing, neuromodulation therapies are valuable albeit invasive. These neuromodulation therapies include spinal cord stimulation.[68] They must be considered after evaluation by a competent neurosurgeon with experience in this field.

Psychotherapeutic Intervention

From the beginning of the condition, the psychological effect of CRPS on the patient must be recognized and addressed. It must be determined whether the psychological distress is secondary to CRPS or whether the patient had preexisting psychological problems that have been aggravated by CRPS.

Because CRPS is a puzzling disease that varies with the patient, many cases have been diagnosed as psychogenic rather than as a medical problem with psychological complications. After a prolonged period of relatively intractable pain, depression can be expected, which will intensify the severity of the symptoms. Psychological guidance and group therapy must accompany psychotherapeutic drugs to enhance the patient's return to meaningful function.

REFERENCES

1. Mersky H, Bogduk N. *Classification of Chronic Pain: Descriptions of Chronic Pain Syndromes and Definition of Pain Terms.* 2nd ed. Seattle, Wash: IASP Press; 1994.

2. Mitchell SW, Morehouse G, Keen WW. *Gunshot Wounds and Other Injuries of the Nerves.* Philadelphia, Pa: JB Lippincott; 1864.

3. Paget J. Clinical lectures on some causes of local paralysis. *Med Times Hosp Gazette.* 1864;1:331.

4. Richards RL. Causalgia: a centennial review. *Arch Neurol.* 1967;16: 339-350.

5. Leriche R. De la causalgic envisage comme une nevrite du sympathique et de son traitement par la denudation et l'excision des plexus nerveux peri-arteriel. *Presse Med.* 1916;24:178-180.

6. Sudeck P. γber die akute (trophoneurotische) Knochenatrophie nach Entzhndungen und Traumen der Extremitten. *Dtsch Med Wochenschr.* 1902:28:336-342.

7. Evans JA. Reflex sympathetic dystrophy. *Surg Clin North Am*. 1946;26: 435–448.

8. Baron R, Levine JD, Fields HL. Causalgia and reflex sympathetic dystrophy: does the sympathetic nervous system contribute to the generation of pain? *Muscle Nerve*. 1999;22:678–695.

9. Bernard C. *An Introduction to the Study of Experimental Medicine*. New York, NY: Dover Publications; 1957.

10. Roberts WJ. A hypothesis on the physiological basis of causalgia and related pains. *Pain*. 1986;24:297–311.

11. Birklein F, Riedl B, Sieweke N, Weber M, Neundorfer B. Neurological findings in complex regional pain syndrome: analysis of 145 cases. *Acta Neurol Scand*. 2000;101:262–269.

12. Blumberg H, Janig W. Clinical manifestations of reflex sympathetic dystrophy and sympathetically maintained pain. In: Wall PD, Melzack R, eds. *Textbook of Pain*. 3rd ed. Edinburgh, Scotland: Churchill Livingstone; 1994.

13. Malecki J, LeBel AA, Bennett GJ, Schwartzman RJ. Patterns of spread in complex regional pain syndrome, type I (reflex sympathetic dystrophy pain). *Pain*. 2000;88:259–266.

14. Stanton-Hicks M, Janig W, Hassenbusch S, Haddox JD, Boas R, Wilson P. Reflex sympathetic dystrophy: changing concepts and taxonomy. *Pain*. 1995;63:127–133.

15. IASP Subcommittee on Taxonomy. Reflex sympathetic dystrophy (1–5). *Pain*. 1986;38(suppl 3):S29–S30.

16. Galer BS, Bruehl S, Harden RN. IASP Diagnostic criteria for complex regional pain syndrome: a preliminary empirical validation study. *Clin J Pain*. 1998;14:48–54.

17. Bruehl S, Harden RN, Galer BS, Saltiz S, Backonja M, Stanton-Hicks M. Complex regional pain syndrome: are there distinct subtypes and sequential stages of the syndrome? *Pain*. 2002;95:119–124.

18. Stanton-Hicks M. Regional anesthetic as a diagnostic tool for CRPS. In: Harden NR, Baron R, Janig W, eds. *Complex Regional Pain Syndrome: Progress in Pain Research and Management*. Vol 22. Seattle, Wash: IASP Press; 2001.

19. Price DD, Bennett GJ, Rafli A. Psychological observations on patients with neuropathic pain relieved by a sympathetic block. *Pain*. 1989;36:273–288.

20. Wasner G, Schattschneider J, Heckman K, Maier C, Baron R. Vascular abnormalities in reflex sympathetic dystrophy (CRPS): mechanisms and diagnostic value. *Brain*. 2001;124:587–599.

21. Stanton-Hicks M, Raj PP, Racz GB. Use of regional anesthetics in the diagnosis of reflex sympathetic dystrophy and sympathetically maintained pain: a critical evaluation. In: Janig W, Stanton-Hicks M, eds. *Reflex*

Sympathetic Dystrophy:A Reappraisal. Progress in Pain Research and Management. Vol 6. Seattle,Wash: IASP Press; 1996.

22. Rauck R. Sympathetic nerve blocks: head, neck and trunk. In: Prithvi RP, ed. *Practical Management of Pain.* 3rd ed. St. Louis, Mo: Mosby; 2000.

23. Cannon WB, Rosenblueth A. *The Supersensitivity of Denervated Structures.* New York, NY: Macmillan Publishing Co Inc; 1949.

24. Axelson J,Thesieff S.A study of supersensitivity in denervated mammalian skeletal muscles. *J Physiol.* 1959;174:178.

25. Fambrough DM, Hartzell HC, Powell JA, Rash JE, Joseph N. *On Differentiation and Organization of the Surface Membrane of a Post-synaptic Cell—The Skeletal Muscle Fiber: Synaptic Transmission and Neuronal Interaction.* New York, NY: Raven Press; 1974.

26. Guth L. 'Trophic' influence of nerve on muscle. *Physiol Review.* 1968;48:645–687.

27. Rosenbleuth A, Luco JV. Study of denervated mammalian skeletal muscle. *Am J Physiol.* 1937;120:781–797.

28. Gunn CC. Causalgia and denervation supersensitivity. *Am J Acupuncture.* 1979;7(4):119–123.

29. Fleming WW,Westfall DP.Adaptive supersensitivity. In:Trendelenberg U, Weiner N, eds. *Handbook of Experimental Pharmacology.* Vol 90, No 1. New York, NY: Springer Publishing Co; 1988.

30. Campbell JN, Meyer RA, Raja SN. Is nociceptor activation by alpha-1 adrenoceptors the culprit in sympathetically-maintained pain? *ASP J.* 1992;1:3–11.

31. Stanton-Hicks M. Complex regional pain syndrome (type I, RSD; type II causalgia): controversies. *Clin J Pain.* 2000;16:S33–S40.

32. Janig W. Organization of the lumbar sympathetic outflow to skeletal muscle and skin of the cat hind limb and tail. *Rev Physiol Biochem Pharmacol.* 1985;102:119–213.

33. Ochoa JL. Reflex? Sympathetic dystrophy? Triple question again. *Mayo Clin Proc.* 1995;70:1124–1126.

34. Torebjork HE,Wahren LK,Wallin G, et al. Noradrenalin-evoked pain in neuralgia. *Pain.* 1995;63:11–20.

35. Schwartzman RJ, McLellan TL. Reflex sympathetic dystrophy: a review. *Arch Neurol.* 1987;44:555–561.

36. Van Der Laan L, Kapitein P,Verhofstad A, Hendriks T, Goris RJ. Clinical signs and symptoms of acute reflex sympathetic dystrophy in one hind limb of the rat, induced by infusion of a free radical donor. *Acta Orthop Belg.* 1998;64:210–217.

37. Birklein F,Weber M, Ernst M, Riedl B, Neundorfer B, Handwerker HO. Experimental tissue acidosis leads to increased pain in complex regional pain syndrome (CRPS). *Pain.* 2000;87:227–234.

38. Van Der Laan L, ter Laak HJ, Gabreels FA, Gabreels F, Goris RJ. Complex regional pain syndrome type I (RSD): pathology of skeletal muscle and peripheral nerve. *Neurology*. 1998;51:20-25.

39. Janig W. CRPS-I and CRPS-II: a strategic view. In: Harden RN, Baron R, Janig W, eds. *Complex Regional Pain Syndromes: Progress in Pain Research and Management.* Vol 22. Seattle, Wash: IASP Press; 2001.

40. Wasner G, Schattschneider J, Heckmann K, Maier C, Baron R. Vascular abnormalities in reflex sympathetic dystrophy (CRPS I): mechanisms and diagnostic value. *Brain*. 2001;124:587-599.

41. Janig W. Pain and the sympathetic nervous system: pathophysiological mechanisms. In: Mathias CJ, Bannister R, eds. *Autonomic Failure*. 4th ed. Oxford, England: Oxford University Press; 1999.

42. Butler SH. Disuse and CRPS. In: Harden RN, Baron R, Janig W, eds. *Complex Regional Pain Syndromes: Progress in Pain Research and Management.* Vol 22. Seattle, Wash: IASP Press; 2001.

43. Hannington-Kiff JG. Does failed opioid modulation in regional sympathetic ganglia cause reflex sympathetic dystrophy? *Lancet*. 1991:338: 1125-1127.

44. Gellman H, Keenan MA, Stone L, Hardy SE, Waters RL, Stewart C. Reflex sympathetic dystrophy in brain-injured patients. *Pain*. 1992;51:307-311.

45. Butler SH, Nyman M, Gordh T. Immobility in volunteers produces signs and symptoms of CRPS(I) and a neglect-like state. *Abstracts of 9th World Congress on Pain*. Seattle, Wash: IASP Press; 1999.

46. Stanos SP, Harden RN, Wagner-Raphael L, Saltz SL. A prospective clinical model for investigating the development of CRPS. In: Harden RN, Baron R, Janig W, eds. *Complex Regional Pain Syndrome: Progress in Pain Research and Management.* Vol 22. Seattle, Wash: IASP Press; 2001.

47. Schattschneider J, Wenzelburger R, Deuschl G, Baron R. Kinetic analysis of the upper extremity in CRPS. In: Harden RN, Baron R, Janig W, eds. *Complex Regional Pain Syndrome: Progress in Pain Research and Management.* Vol 22. Seattle, Wash: IASP Press; 2001.

48. Verdugo RJ, Campero M, Ochoa JL. Phentolamine sympathetic block in painful polyneuropathies: II. Further questioning of the concept of 'sympathetically-maintained pain.' *Neurology*. 1994;4:1010-1014.

49. Bej M, Schwartzmann R. Abnormalities of cutaneous blood flow regulation in patients with reflex sympathetic dystrophy measure by laser Doppler flowmetry. *Arch Neurol*. 1991;48:912-915.

50. Sandrini P. Testing the autonomic nervous system. *IASP Newsletter*. November/December 1998.

51. Cooke ED, Ward C. Vicious circles in reflex sympathetic dystrophy—a hypothesis: discussion paper. *J Roy Soc Med*. 1990;83:96-99.

52. Stanton-Hicks M, Raj PP, Racz GB. Use of regional anesthetics for diagnosis of reflex sympathetic dystrophy and sympathetically maintained pain: a critical evaluation. In: Janig W, Stanton-Hicks M, eds. *Reflex Sympathetic Dystrophy: A Reappraisal: Progress in Pain Research And Management.* Vol 6. Seattle, Wash: IASP Press; 1996.

53. Low PA, Amadio PC, Wilson PR, McManis PG, Willner CL. Laboratory findings in reflex sympathetic dystrophy: a preliminary report. *Clin J Pain.* 1994;10:235–239.

54. Hooshmand H. Is thermal imaging of any use in pain management? *Pain.* 1998;8:166–170.

55. Kingery WS. A critical review of controlled clinical trials for peripheral neuropathic pain and complex regional pain syndromes. *Pain.* 1997;73:123–139.

56. Leitha T, Korpan M, Staudenherz A, Wunderbaldinger P, Fiala V. Five-phase scintography supports the pathophysiological concept of a subclinical inflammatory process in reflex sympathetic dystrophy. *Q J Nucl Med.* 1996;40:188–193.

57. Levine JD, Taiwo YO, Collins SD, Tam JK. Noradrenaline hyperalgesia is mediated through interaction with sympathetic postganglionic neurone terminals rather than activation of primary afferent nociceptors. *Nature.* 1986;323:158–160.

58. Stanton-Hicks M, Baon R, Boas R, et al. Consensus report: complex regional pain syndromes: guidelines for therapy. *Clin J Pain.* 1998;14:155–166.

59. Gullickson G, Licht S. Chapter one definition and philosophy of rehabilitation medicine. In: Licht S, ed. *Rehabilitation and Medicine.* Vol 10. New Haven, Conn: Eliz Licht Publishers; 1968.

60. Lehmann JF, DeLateur BJ. Diathermy and superficial heat, laser and cold therapy. In: Kottke/Lehmann, eds. *Krusen's Handbook of Physical Medicine and Rehabilitation.* 4th ed. Philadelphia, Pa: WB Saunders Co; 1990.

61. Bell KR, Lehmann JF. Effects of cooling on H- and T-reflexes in normal subjects. *Arch Phys Med Rehabil.* 1987;68;490–493.

62. Melzack R, Wall PD. Pain mechanisms: a new theory. *Science.* 1965;150:971–979.

63. Baron R, Schattschneider J, Binder A, Siebrecht D, Wasner G. Relation between sympathetic vasoconstrictor activity and pain and hyperalgesia in complex regional pain syndromes: a case-control study. *Lancet.* 2002;359:1655–1660.

64. Radin EL. The physiology and degeneration of joints. *Sem Arthritis Rheum.* 1972–1973;2:245–257.

65. Geertzen JH, de Bruijn H, de Bruijn-Kofman AT, Arendzen JH. Reflex sympathetic dystrophy: early treatment and psychological aspects. *Arch Phys Med Rehabil.* 1994;75:442-446.

66. Egle UT, Hoffman SO. Psychosomatic aspects of reflex sympathetic dystrophy. In: Stanton-Hicks M, Janig W, Boas RA, eds. *Reflex Sympathetic Dystrophy.* Boston, Mass: Klumer Academic Publishers; 1990.

67. Watson CP, Evans RJ, Watt VR. Post-herpetic neuralgia and topical capsaicin. *Pain.* 1988;33:333-340.

68. Robaina F, Dominguez M, Diaz M, Rodriguez JL, de Vera JA. Spinal cord stimulation for relief of chronic pain in vasospastic disorders of the upper limbs. *Neurosurgery.* 1989;24:63-67.

chapter 12

Rheumatoid Arthritis

In inflammatory joint disease there are 4 major categories to be differentiated: degenerative joint disease, rheumatoid disease, metabolic disorders with articular component, and periarticular conditions.[1] Restriction of motion, swelling, redness, and tenderness, all indicate intra-articular inflammation. The source must be determined.

There are numerous diagnostic procedures that are involved in the differential diagnosis of inflammatory joint disease, and aspiration may be indicated. An elevated synovial fluid leukocyte count indicates possible infection that may require culturing. Evidence of crystals suggests sodium urate or calcium pyrophosphates. A low serum complement suggests rheumatoid arthritis (RA). Once diagnosed, the specific articular pathologic cause must be addressed.

HISTORY

The most devastating and impairing form of articular disease is RA, which poses mandatory rehabilitation efforts from the beginning of the disorder.

Although RA is a rheumatologic disease, it affects joints and musculoskeletal function, which requires medical intervention. It therefore belongs in the category of medical orthopedics. Rheumatoid arthritis is a systemic inflammatory disorder of a chronic nature characterized by a pattern involving synovial joints as well as tendons, ligaments, fascia, and muscles.

The synovial lining of synovial joints is devoid of a basement membrane, which thus permits free diffusion of soluble substances. As synovium lines a closed cavity (synovial joint), any reactive material that enters the joint cavity is difficult to remove. The synovial lining is composed of 2 layers of cells (types A and B) supported by connective tissue. Type A cells are surface pseudopods, with the cytoplasm rich in lysosomes and Golgi complexes. They are phagocytes similar to macrophages. Type B cells are secretory synoreceptor cells containing mostly reticulum and no vacuole or lysosomes.

A typical synovial joint was shown in Figure 1.3 in Chapter 1. The capsule is formed by synovial cells that secrete synovial fluid and is surrounded by a fibrous capsule. The synovium is single cell in content and becomes enlarged and multiplied only when affected by an inflammatory condition.

According to Lee et al,[2] "the pathogenic mechanisms that play a role in inflammatory arthritis such as rheumatoid arthritis remain poorly understood both systemically and in the microenvironment of the diarthrodial joint." Many soluble inflammatory mediators have been identified as being involved in the inflammatory process, but their derivation has remained obscure because studies in humans have been limited and animal studies, as yet, are not productive.

Recent studies using the serum from an engineered mouse model (K/BxN) have cast light on the mechanism of inflammatory hyperplasia and erosive synovitis.[2] The inflammatory agents have included cytokines (interleukin-1), tumor necrosis factor-α (TNF-α), and neutrophils (Figure 12.1). These agents are thought to be manufactured by mast cells, whose activation rapidly releases granules, which in turn release inflammatory factors that invade the synovium. The result is synovitis with all proceeding degrees of damage to the joint.

Historically, mast cells have been implicated in 2 contrasting types of immune responses. First, they can be activated by immunoglobulin IgE receptors to mediate immediate hypersensitivity reactions associated with allergic phenomena. Second, they activate microbial products similar to bacterial infections. With the work of Lee et al[2] and others,[3,4] it becomes apparent that the mast cell is incriminated in the pathogenesis of RA.

Mast cells are considered "sentries" of the immune system, patrolling mucous membranes and other routes of entry. When an antigen appears, the mast cells quickly appear and "dump" their granules filled with histamine and other chemicals, which accounts for the evidence of inflammatory wheals and redness.

Recent evidence points to other causative factors in RA besides mast cells. Wang et al[5] found that binding of immune system lymphocytes to the carbohydrates that weave together with proteins to form cartilage and synovial membranes called *glycosaminoglycans* (GAGs) is involved in RA. Injection of GAGs into the tails of mice caused them to become swollen and red, similar to RA. Upon inspection of these injected tails, thousands of lymphocytes were found in

FIGURE 12.1

Mast Cell Production of Inflammatory Agents Mast cells within blood vessels (BV) extrude through endothelium to penetrate synovial layers of joint. Mast cells then release granules that liberate cytokines and other inflammatory agents, which attack (curved arrows) synovium, causing synovitis.

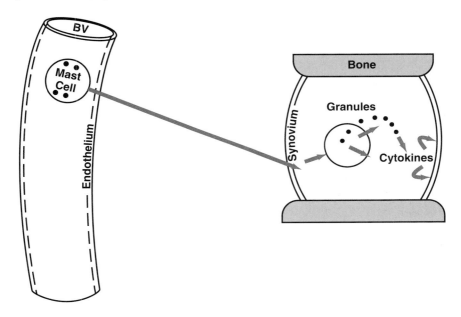

the synovial system attacking the GAGs. Lymphocytes are usually not found in normal synovial fluid.

Glycosaminoglycan-specific lymphocytes were found in bone marrow and not in lymph nodes.[6] This finding indicated a general immune reaction, not merely a local phenomenon, and that the process would continue so long as bone marrow generated the GAG-specific lymphocytes that migrate to the joints.[6] Patients with RA were found to have substantial numbers of GAG-binding cells within the synovial fluid. Why these GAG-specific lymphocytes target carbohydrates rather than proteins remains unclear. Few researchers have studied the biochemistry of carbohydrates and thus have not included carbohydrates in immune reactions but have merely involved proteins and peptides. Now the focus may change.

The combination of mast cell reaction and the carbohydrate linkage portends major advances in acquiring a therapeutic measure that will affect not just the symptoms but also the pathological changes in joint tissues.[6]

DIAGNOSIS

The criteria to diagnose RA is defined by the American Rheumatism Association as:

- morning stiffness,
- pain on motion or tenderness in at least 1 joint,
- swelling of at least 1 joint,
- symmetrical joint swelling with simultaneous involvement of that joint on both sides of the joint,
- subcutaneous nodules on bony prominences on the joint extensor surfaces or in the juxta-articular region,
- radiographic evidence revealing typical changes,
- positive reaction to the agglutination test (rheumatoid factor),
- poor mucin precipitate from synovial fluid, and
- characteristic histologic changes of synovium and of the nodule.

TREATMENT

There are numerous drugs being advocated, which increase as research progress occurs. Many inhibit prostaglandin synthetase activity. These include daily aspirin; nonsteroidal anti-inflammatory drugs (NSAIDs) such as ibuprofen, naproxen, fenoprofen, tolmetin sodium, and sulindac; and cyclooxygenase (COX-2) inhibitors for patients who have stomach sensitivity from NSAIDs.

Systemic steroid therapy has had substantial benefit but with many side effects that are undesirable.

When the above drugs fail to produce a benefit, other medications are indicated. These include gold compounds (thiomalate and thiosulfate), D-penicillamine, and antimalarial drugs such as hydrochloroquine.

There are basic principles that must be addressed in any treatment protocol regarding inflammatory joint disease. Principally, the avoidance of repetitive joint motion minimizes joint stress. The patient must avoid any unnecessary activity and must have structured rest periods between any movement.

Immobilization of an acutely inflamed joint is often indicated but must be carefully controlled to avoid disuse and periarticular contractions. The ergonomics of daily living and work must be carefully evaluated to permit the required functions but with minimal joint stress.

In the acute phase, moist heat is beneficial to decrease inflammation and to permit active motion. The use of cold compresses may be better tolerated by the patient, and it is known that alternating cold and heat has beneficial effect. Both have physiological benefit, so whichever modality is accepted by the patient is the modality indicated.

Because inflammatory joint disease causes diminished muscular activity, atrophy must be minimized. Joint inflammation causes reflex periarticular muscular contraction (known as "spasm") to minimize joint motion. Muscular contraction to minimize atrophy is best done by isometric contraction. This voluntary muscular contraction is without joint motion, whereas isotonic contraction permits and encourages joint motion as well as muscular contraction.

JOINT CONTRACTURE

Any immobilized joint, for whatever reason, tends to develop contracture (shortening) of the fibrous elements of the capsule. This must be minimized by gentle, frequent stretching exercises performed on the patient and by the patient. Again, it must be stated that any exercise—active or passive—is best tolerated by being preceded by heat and followed by cold compresses.

Rheumatoid arthritis is usually manifested by symmetrical joint involvement of the small joints of the feet and hands—the MCP as well as the PIP joints—but also may involve the wrists, elbows, shoulders, knees, and ankles. Essentially, no joint in the body is immune to rheumatoid disease. Because each joint has been addressed in this text, the joints will not be discussed individually here, other than to highlight specifically how RA may differ from other diseases.

Temporomandibular joint involvement in RA, when destructive, poses a substantial impairment, as it impairs mastication and food intake. Cervical spine involvement permits subluxation with potential nerve root or spinal cord entrapment or both. Involvement of the shoulder and elbow impairs placement of the hands and fingers in the needed functional positions.

In the hands, the metacarpal-phalangeal joint is a primary focus of the disease, with frequent subluxations or even total luxations occurring. These joint subluxations involve subluxations of the extensor tendons with rupture of the slips. Splinting is mandated, as is use of dynamic functional orthosis.[6]

OTHER ARTHRITIC CONDITIONS

Osteoarthritis (degenerative joint disease) is a disorder in which the joint narrows and there are bony proliferations at the joint margins. The pathomechanics of this joint deterioration remains unknown. Often osteoarthritis is of only cosmetic concern, because there is no restriction and pain is usually minimal. This is not true of all joints involved, as there is impairment when degeneration occurs in the hip, knee, or first carpometacarpal joint of the hand.

Trauma plays a role in the development of osteoarthritis, as degeneration occurs after damage to the meniscus or the ankle.[7,8] Metabolic arthropathies such as gout usually respond with appropriate medical intervention without degenerative changes.

REFERENCES

1. Swezey RL. Rehabilitation in arthritis and allied conditions. In: Kottke FJ, Lehmann JF, eds. *Krusen's Handbook of Physical Medicine and Rehabilitation*. Philadelphia, Pa: WB Saunders Co; 1990.

2. Lee DM, Friend DS, Gurish MF, Benoist C, Mathis D, Brenner MB. Mast cells: a cellular link between autoantibodies and inflammatory arthritis. *Science*. 2002;297:1689-1692.

3. Echtenacher B, Mannel DN, Hultner L. Critical protective role of mast cells in a model of acute septic peritonitis. *Nature*. 1996;381:75-77.

4. Malaviya R, Ikeda T, Ross E, Abraham SN. Mast cell modulation of neutrophil influx and bacterial clearance at sites of infection through TNF-alpha. *Nature*. 1996;381:77-80.

5. Wang XM, Yuan B, Hou ZL. Role of the deep mesencephalic nucleus in the antinociception induced by stimulation of the anterior pretrecal nucleus in rats. *Brain Res*. 1992;577:321-325.

6. Cailliet R. *Hand Pain and Impairment*. 4th ed. Philadelphia, Pa: FA Davis Co; 1982.

7. Cailliet R. *Knee Pain and Disability*. 3rd ed. Philadelphia, Pa: FA Davis Co; 1992

8. Cailliet R. *Foot and Ankle Pain*. 3rd ed. Philadelphia, Pa: FA Davis Co; 1997.

13

Fibromyalgia

Fibromyalgia syndrome (FMS) is more aptly designated under *rheumatoid disease syndrome,* as designated by the American College of Rheumatology (ACR) in 1990.[1]

HISTORY

Fibromyalgia syndrome was first described in 1816 by William Balfour, a surgeon at the University of Edinburgh. It subsequently was termed chronic rheumatism, myalgia, pressure point syndrome, fibrositis, and myofascial pain syndrome (MPS).

The term *fibromyalgia* is a combination of the Latin words *fibro* (fibrous or connective tissue fibers), *myo* (muscle), and *algia* (pain). *Syndrome* means "a group of signs and/or symptoms of disordered function related to one another by means of some anatomic, physiologic, or biochemical peculiarity. This definition does not include a precise cause of an illness, but does provide a framework of reference for investigating it."[2]

In 1987 the American Medical Association (AMA) recognized fibromyalgia as a true illness and a major cause of impairment and disability.[3] At the second World Congress on Myofascial Pain and Fibromyalgia in Copenhagen in 1992, fibromyalgia was officially recognized as a syndrome, defined as not articular but "the most common cause of chronic widespread musculoskeletal pain."[4] It was subsequently described by van Why[5] as "the presence of an unexplained widespread pain and aching, persistent fatigue, generalized morning stiffness, non-refreshing sleep, and multiple tender points." Van Why stated that patients must have 11 or more tender points for a diagnosis of FMS.[5]

The Copenhagen Declaration added to this definition that, as a syndrome, fibromyalgia encompassed headaches, irritable bladder, dysmenorrhea, cold sensitivity, Raynaud phenomenon, restless legs, atypical patterns of numbness and tingling, exercise intolerance, and complaints of weakness. The Copenhagen Declaration also attributed the symptoms of depression and anxiety in patients with FMS as a result and not the cause of the condition.[3]

To fit the syndrome's definition, the pain that results from pressing on the tender points must be local and not referred. It was also required by the Copenhagen Declaration that tender points be present in all 4 quadrants of the body—both upper extremities and both lower extremities—and have been continuous—albeit fluctuating from day to day—for at least 3 months. In addition to the 18 tender points specified by the Copenhagen Declaration, tender spots are usually found in the neck and at the base of the skull (Figure 13.1).

Today, the diagnosis of FMS remains unclear and even unaccepted— sometimes called merely another chronic pain syndrome—because there are currently no laboratory tests that confirm the diagnosis.

The myofascia is a thin, almost transparent tissue that layers the muscle fibers, giving that specific muscle its shape. This layer apparently contains neurotransmitters, which are nerve end-organs that, when inflamed or irritated, transmit impulses that ascend C fibers and A-alpha fibers to convey the sensation of pain.

Fascia contains a ground substance, a semisolid or fluid gelatinous substance that was described by Butler.[6] "The tiniest muscle fiber is wrapped with fascia. . . . [A]s the fiber ends the fascia continues until it attaches to the bone (periosteum) as a tendon." When the fascia is strained, it undergoes chemical changes.

In his classic text on the management of pain, Bonica[7] devoted merely 1 page to the syndrome, which he called *primary fibromyalgia syndrome*. He quoted the International Association for the Study of Pain (IASP) Committee on Taxonomy as stating: "The condition is defined as diffuse, aching musculoskeletal pain associated with multiple discrete predicable tender points and stiffness."

Bonica[7] further stated:

> The most important feature of fibromyalgia syndrome is widespread aching of more than 3 months duration that is poorly circumscribed and perceived as deep, usually referred to muscle or bony prominences. Although pain in the trunk and proximal girdle is aching in character, distal limb pain is often perceived as associated with fatigue, swelling, numbness, or stiff feeling. The pain is usually continuous, but there can be day-to-day fluctuation in pain intensity and shifts from one area to another. Stiffness, which is perceived as an increased resistance to joint movement, particularly towards the end of range of movement, is worse in the mornings. . . . The

FIGURE   13.1

Location of Tender Spots in Fibromyalgia Location of tender points found in FMS, front and back.

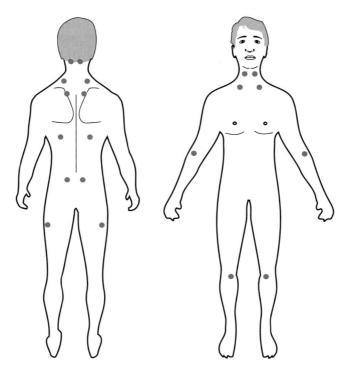

patient complains of fatigue and even exhaustion . . . often associated with disturbed, restless sleep. Trigger points or discrete local areas of deep tenderness involving a variety of otherwise normal tissues are a pathognomonic feature provided that at least 12 are present.

All these symptoms are subjective and vague, which makes the diagnosis of the syndrome difficult. Even trigger points are not specific, because the individuals who administer these tests may vary as to intensity or area of pressure. Although no specific test has been confirmed, Bengtsson and Bengtsson[8] noted that, in 8 patients with characteristic symptoms of FMS who received regional sympathetic blockade with bupivacaine, the number of tender points markedly diminished and rest pain significant decreased compared with patients receiving sham injections.

MYOFASCIAL TRIGGER POINTS

Because trigger points play such a vital role in MPS, they merit careful examination. They are the hallmark of identification of MPS. To add to the confusion of terms, Starlanyl and Copeland[9] in their classic text, *Fibromyalgia and Chronic Myofascial Pain Syndrome: A Survival Manual*, state: "Trigger points can be present as single points, multiple trigger points, as a part of chronic MPS, or as a part of the FMS/MPS Complex. . . . Note that trigger points are 'not' part of FMS. . . . [I]ndividual [trigger points] can but do not always go on to become chronic MPS which can, but does not always become FMS/MPS Complex." Someone wishing to fully understand what a trigger point objectively is can be confused by these comments.

Starlanyl and Copeland[9] continue, "Trigger points can be felt as painful lumps of hardened fascia, possibly due to constriction of blood and other fluids. When a nerve passes through a muscle between ropy bands they are called [trigger point] 'nerve entrapment.' No two patients' problems are exactly alike . . . and can vary from hour to hour and day to day."

Carol Warfield[10] in her text, *Principles and Practice of Pain Management*, devotes a chapter on myofascial syndrome but prefaces her comments with "unfortunately, it is poorly defined, nebulous, and masked by various guises." Other authors wrote: "The hallmark of identification of the myofascial syndrome is the trigger points,"[11] but the histological evidence from Starlanyl and Copeland[9] is controversial. According to Wolfe, the trigger points "are supposedly characteristic on several counts: they are remarkably constant anatomically"[12] and occur only in certain areas of the musculoskeletal topography. "This constancy is considered to be a factor that sustains the veracity of the syndrome."[13]

Stimulation of the trigger point by pressure or electrical current produces a characteristic radiation of pain that is not anatomically radicular but is consistent. This pain has been clearly delineated by Simons[11] and Travell and Rinzler.[14]

The syndrome is currently divided into 2 types: primary and secondary. Primary MPS is the result of direct trauma usually to a muscle.[15] This trauma may be due to repetitive strain or sprain, postural, lifting, or direct impact. Secondary MPS is focal muscle involvement occurring from an incident outside the muscle, such as a herniated disk or articular disease.

In an article in the *Journal of Musculoskeletal Pain*, Walen et al[16] stated that "the multifaceted expression of FMS, along with unpredictable treatment outcomes, has led a number of researchers to propose that FMS may not be a single disease, and/or that subgroups of FMS patients may be identifiable." According to Turk and Flor[17] in an article in the *Journal of Rheumatology*, "this suggests that treatment efficacy may depend on identifiable patient characteristics."

The identified subgroups ("clusters") of patients with FMS are as follows:

- *dysfunctional,* characterized by high levels of pain, disability, and psychological distress;
- *interpersonally distressed,* characterized by interpersonal difficulties and low levels of social support; and
- *adaptive copers,* characterized by low distress and disability and high levels of self-sufficiency.

These clusters essentially relate to patients suffering from any neuromusculoskeletal pain syndrome, so they do not clearly characterize 3 variants of FMS. The conclusion by Walen and coworkers[16] was that there was no evidence that intervention differentially affected the clusters.

CAUSE OF FMS

The true cause of FMS is not known or fully accepted, and the microscopic examinations of the affected muscles and trigger points are probably the result of the condition rather than the cause.

A neurologic basis has been proposed in which the increased autonomic tone in the area of the trigger point causes vasoconstriction with buildup of metabolites that irritate the nerve endings, resulting in pain.[10] This results in a reverberating cycle not much different than in complex regional pain syndrome. A relationship to that condition has been previously mentioned, and the treatment protocol for FMS is not substantially different from those for CRPS.

DIAGNOSIS

The history of generalized muscular pains, localized tender spots, and resultant fatigue indicates the possibility of FMS. A finding of the correct percentage of trigger points in the anatomical locations is considered *the* diagnostic feature that confirms the diagnosis. Findings of these triggers and the radiating pattern of pain are consistent with FMS. Elimination of these trigger points by injection of a local anesthetic agent confirms the diagnosis.

The classic sites of these triggers are also diagnostic: 2 in the neck (the superior aspect of the sternocleidomastoid and the scalene muscles), the middle portion of the superior aspect of the trapezius muscle, the rhomboid muscle (just inferior to the 12th rib at the lateral aspect of the paraspinous muscle mass), and in the center of the musculus gluteus maximus (Figure 13.1).

TREATMENT

Treatment cannot be specified as acute or chronic as there are no specified stages of the syndrome and all symptoms and findings may be present or just a few, which is what is perplexing about the syndrome. Treatment is aimed at alleviating the symptoms, decreasing their severity, and preventing disability rather than attempting to remove or modify the pathology, which is not currently recognized.

As in any chronic pain syndrome, reassurance of the patient is mandatory. The "disease" is not life-threatening; nor does it permanently damage tissues or cause structural damage. Its duration will be modified by the patient's willingness to tolerate pain by realizing that "hurt" is not "harm."

Passive Treatment

Passive treatment implies treatment administered "to" the patient. To alleviate the tenderness and pain of the trigger points, local injections with an analgesic agent may be helpful.[18-20] There is controversy regarding this procedure. Some claim that local mechanical damage to the muscle tissue from the needle and the chemical injected may damage the microfibrillar structures of the muscle.[18] Ischemia has been proposed as a mediator of pain from chemical inflammation at the nerve endings, so an injection can cause vasodilatation, which is therapeutic.

Trigger points can be addressed by spray therapy (ethyl chloride) to the palpable points, which "refrigerates" the tissues. Deep friction massage to the points preceded by the application of ice packs and followed by heat packs are also of value.

With the joints showing some restriction and loss of range of motion, manipulation and/or mobilization has value.

Active Therapy

Active therapy refers to treatment done "by" the patient, albeit with assistance and guidance by a therapist as well as self-performed. Flexibility exercises are the key as patients with this syndrome tend to acquire limited range of motion due to contracture of collagen fibers in connective tissues. There are numerous forms of flexibility exercises, but currently the trend toward Pilates-based body conditioning seems sensible as the exercises are concerned with flexibility as well as coordination with no attempt at muscle resistance.

Aerobic exercises are beneficial and must be carefully moderated by the physician so that the exercises are not too aggressive or aggravating, as they can discourage the patient from maximum effort.

Strengthening exercises are also desireable as weakness is a frequent complaint. Strengthening exercises must be done slowly and gradually so as not to cause symptoms of soreness or aching.

Medication

Salicylates are of value and are usually tolerated well. Nonsteroidal anti-inflammatory drugs (NSAIDs) also have value in decreasing pain. Antispasmodics (such as diazepam or carisoprodol) have been advocated, as the condition seems to have a "spasm" component. Unfortunately, antispasmodic drugs have a central effect that causes depression, which is so prevalent in patients with FMS. Antidepressants are valuable, because they combat this depression and decrease the severity of pain.

Psychotherapeutic Approach

As there is a large psychogenic component to FMS, early psychological intervention is suggested, with cognitive therapy being the most productive.[21]

REFERENCES

1. Wolfe F, Smythe A, Yunis MB, et al. The American College of Rheumatology 1990 Criteria for the Classification of Fibromyalgia: report of the Multicenter Criteria Committee. *Arthritis Rheum.* 1990;33:160–172.

2. Thomas CL, ed. *Taber's Cyclopedic Medical Dictionary.* 16th ed. Philadelphia, Pa: FA Davis; 1989.

3. Smythe HA. Non articular rheumatism. In: *Arthritis and Allied Conditions.* 10th ed. McCarty DJ, ed. Philadelphia, Pa: Lea and Febiger; 1985.

4. Myopain '92: abstracts from the 2nd World Congress on Myofascial Pain and Fibromyalgia, Copenhagen, Denmark, August 17–20, 1992. *Scand J Rheumatol.* 1992;94:1–70.

5. Rubin D. An approach to the management of myofascial trigger point syndromes. *Arch Phys Med Rehabil.* 1981;62:107–110.

6. Butler S. *Conquering Carpal Tunnel Syndrome and Other Repetitive Strain Injuries.* Oakland, Calif: New Harbinger Publications; 1996.

7. Bonica JJ. *The Management of Pain.* 2nd ed. Vol 1. Philadelphia, Pa: Lea & Febiger; 1990.

8. Bengtsson A, Bengtsson M. Regional sympathetic blockade in primary fibromyalgia. *Pain.* 1988;33:61.

9. Starlanyl D, Copeland ME. *Fibromyalgia and Chronic Myofascial Pain Syndrome: A Survival Manual.* Oakland, Calif: New Harbinger Publications; 1996.

10. Warfield CA. *Principles and Practice of Pain Management.* New York, NY: McGraw-Hill; 1993.

11. Wolfe F. Fibrosis, fibromyalgia, and musculoskeletal disease: the current status of the fibrositis syndrome. *Arch Phys Med Rehabil.* 1988;69: 527–531.

12. Rogers EJ, Rogers R. Fibromyalgia and myofascial pain: either, neither or both? *Orthop Rev.* 1989;18:1217–1224.

13. Simons DG. Myofascial trigger point: a need for understanding. *Arch Phys Med Rehabil.* 1981;62:97–99.

14. Travell JG, Rinzler SG. The myofascial genesis of pain. *Postgrad Med.* 1952; 11:425.

15. Yunis MB, Kalyan-Raman UP, Kalyan-Raman K. Primary fibromyalgia syndrome and myofascial pain: clinical features and muscle pathology. *Arch Phys Med Rehabil.* 1988;69:451–454.

16. Walen HR, Cronan TA, Serber ER, Groessl E, Oliver K. Subgroups of fibromyalgia patients: evidence for heterogeneity and an examination of differential effects following a community-based intervention. *J Musculoskeletal Pain.* 2002;10:9–32.

17. Turk DC, Flor H. Primary fibromyalgia is greater than tender points: towards a multiaxial taxonomy. *J Rheumatol*. 1989;16(suppl 19):80–86.

18. Garvey TA, Marks MR, Wiesel SW. A prospective, randomized, double-blind evaluation of trigger-point injection therapy for low back pain. *Spine*. 1989;14:962–964.

19. Loeser JD, ed. *Bonica's Management of Pain*. 3rd ed. Philadelphia, Pa: Lippincott, Williams & Wilkins; 2003.

20. Tarsy JM. *Pain Syndromes and their Treatment*. Springfield, Ill: CC Thomas; 193.

21. Beck JS. *Cognitive Therapy*. New York, NY: Guilford Press; 1995.

INDEX

α-blockers to treat neuropathic pain in CRPS, 186
γ-aminobutric acid (GABA) to treat neuropathic pain in CRPS, 186

A

Achilles tendinitis
  bursae inflamed concurrent with, 133
  diagnosis of, 131
  history of, 131
  treatment of, 132
Achilles tendon tear, history, diagnosis, and treatment of, 132
Acromioclavicular (AC) joint pain, 86–89
  diagnosis of, 87–89
  history of, 86
  treatment of, 89
Active should exercises, 91
Acute pain
  cause of, 155, 159
  healing process for, 160
Adhesive capsulitis, inflammation leading to, 82
Adhesive tendinitis, 121–122
Allodynia
  ice and heat to relieve, 185
  myelinated A beta nerve fibers transmitting, 175, 176
  spreading patterns of, 177
Analgesic agent, injection of
  CRPS treated using, 182
  degenerative arthritis treated using, 56
  dislocation of AC joint treated using, 89
  fibromyalgia treated using, 204
  heel spur treated using, 134
  pain and impairment of cervical spine treated using, 50
  patellofemoral pain syndromes treated using, 145–146
  trigger fingers treated using, 122
Ankle
  first-, second-, and third-degree sprains of, 129–131
  involvement in rheumatoid arthritis of, 197
Annular fibers
  disk degeneration involving damage to, 53
  dislocation of radial head within, 107
  rotational forces tearing disk, 40–42
  torn in whiplash injury, 58
Annulus, 26–28
  collagen fibers in, 27

Anticonvulsants to treat neuropathic pain in CRPS, 186
Antimalarial drugs in treatment of rheumatoid arthritis, 196
Antispasmodics to treat fibromyalgia, 205
Arachnoiditis, 172
Arm movement, planes of, 79
Arthritis, degenerative. See Osteoarthritis
Arthritis, rheumatoid. See Rheumatoid arthritis (RA)
Aspirin in treatment of rheumatoid arthritis, 196
Autonomic nervous system (ANS)
  components of, 180
  in CRPS, 169–170
  sympathetic and parasympathetic systems in, 174

B

Biceps mechanisms, 87
Bier blocks to treat pain in CRPS, 186–187
Biopsychosocial aspects of low back pain, 30
  aggravation of condition by, 47
  fatigue one of, 43, 44
  fear one of, 43, 44
Brachial muscle activating flexion of elbow complex, 102
Brain infarct, CRPS occurring following, 165
Bucket tear of meniscus, 145
Bunion
  diagnosis of, 137
  history of, 136
  treatment of, 137–138
Bursitis, posterior calcaneal, 132–133

C

Calcaneal spurs
  diagnosis of, 133–134
  history of, 133
  treatment of, 134
Calcaneofibular ligament, incidence of injury to, 129
Calmoudin activity in progressive scoliosis, 69
Cannon's law, 35–36, 168
Capsaicin, topical, to treat CRPS, 186
Carpal tunnel syndrome (CTS)
  diagnosis of, 114–115
  history of, 113
  incidence of, 113
  treatment of, 115–116

Beyond Gross Anatomy

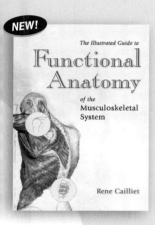

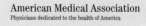